GU01017789

A Mind To

A Personal Search For Therapy

Polly Fielding

www.pollyfielding.com

Copyright © 2013 Polly Fielding

All rights reserved.

ISBN:1482656574
ISBN-13: **978-1482656572**

All rights reserved, no part of this publication may be
reproduced by any means, electronic, mechanical, or
photocopying, documentary, film or otherwise without prior
permission of the author.

Also by Polly Fielding:

And This Is My Adopted Daughter
*The powerful true story of an adopted child's
relationship with two mothers*

Crossing The Borderline
Inside a therapeutic community

Letting Go
A trilogy comprising the current book plus the two
above

The 5:2 Diet Made eZy
A proven, painless way to lose weight

The 5:2 Vegetarian Diet Made eZy
The veggie version

Missing Factor
A personal experience of haemophilia

Going In Seine
An apartment in Paris? A crazy idea!

Cover art by the author

To Rai, for keeping his promise

Author's Note

Anyone who has read my book "And This Is My Adopted Daughter" will understand how my deeply unhappy childhood in my adoptive family left me severely scarred emotionally and in need of therapy.

Preface

Signs of serious disturbance were present from the age of twelve when I secretly cut myself in an attempt to express the terrible rejection I felt when my parents adopted another baby. I was convinced that I wasn't good enough for them. Perhaps they hoped that the next child would prove more acceptable.

Desperate for my parents' attention I tried everything I could to please, annoy or upset them. My behaviour resulted in beatings from my father and daily scorn and contempt from my mother. Nothing I could do was ever right. I gradually accepted that I was useless, stupid and unlovable. This message seemed to be reinforced by the nuns at school who indoctrinated me with the belief that I was worthless unless every second of my life was spent selflessly in the service of others.

My need for therapy surfaced after an overdose when I was twenty-one. A session with a psychiatrist at that point began many years seeking the treatment that could help me to think more positively about myself.

My mother always maintained that my unhappiness was my 'imagination.' My parents never visited me in hospital, sent a card or even once asked me how I was feeling. I was a disgrace to the family and now there was no hope that I could match up to my older sister, their natural daughter. And tracing my birth mother was the ultimate sin, which resulted in exclusion from the family inheritance. For me this spelt total rejection.

I have spent much of my adult life trying to help myself and get therapy for my problems. But the workings of the mind are still a mystery. Progress in this area is slow. We can transplant hearts but we can't mend them.

I've tried many different types of therapy but none has provided the solution I am looking for, perhaps because the answers lie somewhere within me. Each treatment held, in the beginning, a promise of recovery but before long disillusionment and disappointment set in. My expectations were too high and I always viewed therapy as something that was being done to me to make me better. I needed to realise that unless I took responsibility and became an active participant in the process no therapy, however good, would be effective.

My story about my search for the right sort of help is far from unique. There are lots of us who suffer, our hurt invisible to those around us. An emotional disability, unlike a physical one, cannot be seen. I felt I had to keep my hurt hidden, my feelings of isolation, neediness, despair…locked away where no one knew about them. I tried to look smiling, confident, happy so that people would like me. And sometimes it worked… but when the effort became too great my defences failed completely and I was forced to admit defeat.

I quickly discovered the stigma that mental health problems carry. On many occasions I've feared that someone would find out about my breakdowns or realise that I was attending sessions with a mental health professional. I knew that if the truth were known, my teaching job would be in jeopardy; after all nobody wants a loony in charge of a class of children, do they? So I carefully guarded my dark secret but lived with the fear of discovery and the shame it would bring.

This book is in part an attempt to break my taboo of talking about my emotional problems; it also shows the minefield that is the world of therapy. Names of all healthcare professionals and patients have been changed to protect their identities.

Polly Fielding

Chapter One

"Get out! Go and live with whoever you want! And don't ever set foot in this house again!"

I cringe from Mummy's fury over my decision to move into a school colleague's flat, a short bus ride away.

I returned from college intending to live at home. I don't want to leave but I can't tolerate rules that might be appropriate if I were fourteen but not now I'm a twenty-one year-old teacher. I spent three years at college. And during the first year I obeyed Mummy's three parting commandments: Thou shalt not drink. Thou shalt not smoke. Thou shalt not date boys. Then a priest told me in Confession that she was being too hard on me. He gave me the Go Ahead I needed to try to lead some sort of independent existence; though the guilt remains and holding hands is as far as I dare go with any boyfriend.

My current boyfriend, who's Indian, isn't allowed near the house. Mummy's never wanted to meet him. I didn't realise until I showed her a photograph of him that she was prejudiced against coloured people.

I'm forbidden to smoke at home, even though Daddy does, and if I'm five minutes later than the midnight curfew it's regarded as blatant disobedience. To stay here means I'll never get the chance to find out who I am, have the freedom to live my own life in my own way.

Although Claire has warned me that the place isn't up to much, I'm unprepared for the tiny, squalid premises above the dry cleaner's. It consists of two bedrooms and a kitchen. There's a toilet and bath in an unheated outbuilding in the back alley.

The door to Claire's room doesn't close properly. I turn up the radio in an effort to drown out the sounds of lovemaking. Sex was never discussed at home. At twenty-one, still a virgin, I'm shocked at Claire's promiscuity. But I feel sorry and somehow responsible for her.

Claire is two years older than me. Her mother died when she was eighteen. She hates her father, a strict disciplinarian, and seeks love and attention from any man she meets. She doesn't care about herself. Perhaps I can help her.

This morning she was sick. She sat chain-smoking, ashen-faced, watching me eat breakfast.

"Claire, what's up? Are you ill?" I was genuinely concerned about her.

"No… I'm three months pregnant." She looked utterly hopeless.

I was stunned. "Are you sure?"

She nodded.

"Who's the father?"

"I don't know. I think it may be the lorry driver I went out with a couple of times." He was the bastard who had broken her nose. I'd taken her to hospital that night.

I've come back late tonight having spent, as usual, as much time as possible away from this place. I know from the silence and Claire's open door that she has no visitor.

Normally we chat. But I can see immediately that something is terribly wrong.

Claire is slumped on her bed, her face pale, expressionless.

"What's the matter, Claire?"

No answer.

"Claire, please talk to me."

Her gaze remains fixed, her eyes glazed.

Panic stirs in the pit of my stomach.

"Claire, what have you done? I have to know."

"I've taken some tablets." Her tone is flat, lifeless.

"What tablets? How many? When?" I fire questions like bullets. I've no idea what I'm going to do.

"I don't know how many. I crushed them up in a milky drink," she says tonelessly.

I rush to the kitchen. In the bin is an empty painkiller bottle.

I hurry back to Claire's bedroom. Her eyes are half-closed.

"Claire. I've got to call an ambulance."

"No… You're not to do anything. Just leave me alone."

"I *can't*. You might die. I've kept everything you've told me secret but I can't just sit here and do nothing."

I can see she's angry. But I run down the metal stairs to the nearest phone box and dial 999, my hands shaking.

"She's taken an overdose and she's pregnant," I tell the ambulance man.

They're going to keep her in hospital. I can't go back to the flat. I ring a friend, explain what's happened and ask to stay the night.

It takes an hour to reach my friend's home in London. Her mother is kind. She makes me a meal and the three of us talk about Claire.

"I'm going to help her bring up the baby," I tell them.

"Polly, you can't do that. You have your own life to think about. You'll have to tell her tomorrow that you've thought it over and you've changed your mind."

They're right. But I don't know how I'm going to do it. How can I face Claire and tell her I can't keep my promise? That she will have to manage alone?

*

Claire rang me at school again today. Without speaking I replaced the receiver.

I haven't got the courage to tell her our friendship is over, that I never want to see her again. I shared her problems from the moment I moved in with her, agonised over her pregnancy, tried mediate between her and her father. I lost myself completely in her life, her traumas.

My visit to the maternity ward ended my involvement. I watched Claire holding hands with her new partner, felt an overwhelming surge of pity for her tiny daughter in the crib, left quickly and ran outside to the bus stop, feeling confused and angry.

*

With nowhere else to go I'm back home. I have no one to confide in. Daddy sits in front of the TV every evening while Mummy reads the newspaper. Neither of them notices I'm constantly on the verge of tears. I hate them and I hate myself. I'm pathetic, wrapped up in self-pity, scared to go out. I'm desperate to escape – but to where? I'm no use to myself or anyone else. I don't know who I am or what I want.

My Indian boyfriend is still banned from our house. The relationship is just about over anyway. The more I wander aimlessly round the house the greater my desperation. I've tried so hard to concentrate on something, *anything*. Anxiety is building within me. My chest is getting tighter. I can hardly breathe. I've reached screaming pitch. I can't take any more.

This is how it is. This is how it's going to be. Nothing's going to change...

On impulse I take a bottle of aspirin and a glass of water to my bedroom.

I tip some tablets into my hand. They'll make the pain disappear. I must get rid of the hurt. I cup my hand to my mouth then quickly swallow a few mouthfuls of water to wash away the bitter taste.

That wasn't so difficult.

The second handful goes down more easily. I lie on the bed to see what effect they will have...

I took the tablets at eight o'clock. It's now a quarter past. The pain hasn't lessened so I'll take some more. I just want to feel better…

I'm not sure how long I've been lying here staring at the red flowers on the curtains. The numbers on the clock are blurry, my head is fuzzy. The tightness across my chest has gone. It's like I'm not really here. I can't feel my body. There's a buzzing in my ears.

I close my eyes. No thoughts, no emotions…

*

A sudden familiar noise: my alarm has gone off. It's daylight.

I don't understand what's happening. My head aches dreadfully. I'm icy cold and lying fully dressed on my bed. Why didn't I get undressed last night?

The half-empty bottle on my bedside table jogs my memory. I drag myself to the bathroom, splash my face with water. The mirror shows red-rimmed eyes like I've been crying. I mustn't let Mummy see me close up.

I can't eat breakfast; the sight of it makes my stomach heave.

I grab my coat and pull it closely round me. I'm shivering as I push my moped out of the garage. It's like I'm riding to school in a dream. Nothing looks real…

I park the machine close to the school entrance, trying to act as normal, hoping to avoid the other teachers. But the Headmaster is in the corridor approaching me, a concerned expression on his face.

"Polly, you don't look well. Whatever's the matter?"

I can't speak, can't prevent the tears overflowing.

He gestures to his office. "Come in and sit down. Tell me about it," he says gently.

I follow him meekly, not knowing what else to do.

"I've noticed you've not been your normal, cheerful self since Claire left," he begins sympathetically.

From somewhere far off I hear myself pouring out the story about Claire. I tell him everything that happened, how devastating it was for me too…

"And I took a load of aspirin last night." This last sentence has a dull, monotonous quality to it.

He reacts instantly, alarm filling his eyes.

"Come on. We've got to get you to the hospital." He takes me by the arm, guides me to his car then goes back indoors for a few moments to make arrangements for the supervision of my class…

He's chatting as he drives. I can't take in what he's saying, picking out only a few odd words here and there.

He parks the car outside Casualty. He helps me out, leads me into the white-walled entrance where he speaks quietly to a nurse in a blue uniform.

She takes me to a small cubicle. The doctor comes in drawing the curtain behind him.

I'm frightened. They look severe and have brought in some nasty-looking equipment.

"What are you going to do?" I ask. My voice is trembling. Surely they can see I'm scared.

They make no attempt to reassure me.

"Right. It'll probably make no difference now but we're going to wash your stomach out," the doctor states coldly.

Pushing me back onto the bed, the nurse thrusts a piece of thick, cold tubing inside my mouth.

"Keep your mouth open! Swallow this!"

Terrified, I do as she says. The tube sticks in my throat. I try to tell them it's too big but she's repeating, "Swallow it!"

I can't stop gagging as the hard rubber scrapes against the sides of my throat. It's being pushed further and further down. There's a funnel attached to the top of it. She pours liquid into it. My stomach is filling up. I'm going to burst...

A sudden pull and the tube slithers out of my body. I heave.

The nurse turns me onto my side. I throw up violently into the bucket on the floor beside the bed.

I've never been so sick. My eyes are blurred with tears. There's a disgusting taste in my mouth and the rubber stinks. I'm still heaving.

The doctor gives me a rough paper towel to wipe away the vomit dripping from my mouth.

"Perhaps *that* will teach you not to waste our time," he says harshly.

No one understands. No one cares. I might as well be dead...

I've never been to a psychiatrist before.

My doctor referred me after the overdose. "He'll sort you out," he told me confidently.

I'm on time for my ten o'clock appointment. The school Christmas holidays have begun so no one will know I've been here. I'd be too ashamed.

People only see a psychiatrist when they're crazy, don't they? I'm just miserable, fed up with life…

The clinic looks like a small hospital. I go to Reception from where an old lady shows me into the psychiatrist's room. He's sitting behind a desk. His black hair streaked with grey, he's peering at me over the top of his glasses.

"Do sit down," he says, glancing at the paperwork in front of him.

I perch nervously on the edge of the chair, directly facing him.

He comes straight to the point: "Why did you take an overdose?"

He's asked me in the same way that Mummy used to question me. I begin to say, "I...don't know…" then realise I'm responding like a naughty child. I've got to speak. The question needs an answer but it has to be the right one. If I keep quiet I'll be in trouble. But if I don't give the correct answer he'll react badly…

If I don't talk soon he's going to get cross with me. My mind's blank. I look up at him, waiting. Can't he see by my eyes how desperately unhappy I am?

Covering my face with my hands I begin to cry – and I can't stop crying. I try to talk but there's a big lump in my throat; my head is too fuzzy.

He watches me for what seems like ages.

"I think what you need is a few days' rest in hospital," he says eventually. He pauses from writing on a sheet of paper. "Er… have you got a friend who could take you to Shenley Hospital? It's best to go by car – difficult to get to by bus."

I nod. I'm still crying as I dial the Headmaster's number. He gave it to me before school finished, saying he and his wife were willing help me in any way they could.

I wait outside the clinic. They're coming immediately.

I sit in the corridor, head down…

The Headmaster's wife introduces herself and asks for my address. They are taking me to collect my nightwear, toiletries and a change of clothes for my stay.

The car stops outside my parents' house.

Whatever is Mummy going to say? She didn't even know I was going to see a psychiatrist.

"We'll wait here for you. Don't rush."

I go into the kitchen. Mummy is cooking.

"Where've you been? You didn't say you were going out. Dinner's nearly ready."

"I'm not having dinner – I'm going to Shenley Hospital," I say quietly.

"*You're going where*?" She's agitated.

I wince.

"I've been to see a psychiatrist and he says I've got to go in for a rest. Will you come and visit me?" I sound like a small child. I can't help it. I want her to see how distressed I am...

She doesn't look at me. She's taking the potatoes to the sink to drain them.

"It's all in your mind!" she exclaims bitterly. "You've been telling people lies about us. You think I don't know? Don't expect any sympathy from us! Of course we won't come and see you! You've been nothing but trouble since the day we adopted you."

I'm heartbroken. I run to my room, throw some things into a bag, head for the waiting car.

We don't talk during the half-hour drive through the countryside. I'm crying but there are no tears.

We park outside a low, grim-looking building with narrow windows. Inside, the green-painted brick walls stretch a long way. At the end is a room like a doctor's surgery.

"We'll come and see you," the Headmaster promises kindly.

I want to beg them to take me back with them. I can't stay here where nobody knows or understands me. But they've gone.

"Get undressed and step on the scales," a nurse says severely. She chats to another nurse about what they're going to do in their free time. She ignores me...

After taking my personal details the nurse ushers me into a room with seats round the edge. I'm wearing my night-clothes. There are about ten women sitting here. Everyone is ready for bed, like me. But it's only three o'clock. I feel bewildered, lost. What am I supposed to do?

I can see by their faces that no one wants to talk. And I don't either...

I start to cry openly. I don't care who sees me now. If I stay my mind will be dead like these patients. No one seems to notice me here. It's like I'm invisible.

"There's a phone call for you," a nurse tells me.

"Polly, what are you doing in a place like that?" It's Rita, my older sister. She sounds surprised, shocked.

"I'm not well," I reply feebly.

"Look, staying there isn't going to help you. Let me come over and get you. You can come with Mike and me and the baby tonight to Mike's parents in Cumbria."

I know I'll be unhappy if I go with them and that will make everyone around me depressed too.

"No, I'll stay here," I tell her.

"It's up to you. But if you change your mind, tell me," she says crisply. She gives me her in-laws' number.

*

I can't eat the unpleasant-looking food on the trolley. Instead of joining the other patients at the table I go to the bed I've been allocated in the ward.

I lie sobbing for what must be hours. Nobody comes to me. Nobody asks what's wrong.

I look at my watch. Eight o'clock: too late to ring Rita now. She'll have left. But I'll phone first thing in the morning. Somehow I'll find my way to the Lake District. It has to be better than staying here, forgotten about by everyone.

Chapter Two

I have decided to start a new life in another country.

When Mummy showed me the advertisement for teachers in Ontario, Canada, I knew I could leave with her blessing. Sharing a flat close to home was an insult it seemed, but going to another country to live met with her approval. And anything I did only felt right to me if it was acceptable to Mummy. Even at twenty-three I longed for her to be proud of me, to love me as I felt she loved Rita, her natural daughter.

Determined to make her and Daddy proud of me I boarded the liner, *The Empress of Canada*, at Liverpool. I waved to Daddy until he became a tiny dot on the quayside grateful that he, at least, had come to see me off. I left full of hope that finally I could break free from the unhappiness within me.

But feeling lost and childlike, I fell out with my flatmates and work colleagues within weeks. I tried desperately to get on with them but they didn't appear to like me. Whatever I did always annoyed those around me. But nobody bothered to explain why. Feeling totally rejected, I moved out to rent a place on my own.

I loved my job, got on well with the eight to ten year old children in my class. If they liked me how come people of my own age did not?

I confided in the Principal about my unhappy childhood in a family where I felt sure my adopted parents loved their own daughter better than me, despite everything I did to try to please them. I told her of my distress when they adopted Teresa when I was twelve years old, how I felt they were trying to replace me because I wasn't good enough.

Sister Carla Marie seemed to understand my unhappiness. "I think I hate my mother," I told her. She nodded sympathetically. I even told her how guilty I felt when I let my boyfriend touch my breasts. "Can't you ever forgive yourself?" She asked. But Mummy, Daddy and the Catholic Church required me to be perfect in every thought, word and deed. Each failing was yet another sin to be declared in Confession in church, in order to be forgiven by God. There was no excuse for giving in to my sexual desires in any way.

Sister feels sorry for me. She was the one I rang when I overdosed just before Christmas. Had she not taken me from my attic apartment to the Emergency Room I would have died. She agreed not to tell the rest of the staff what I'd done but to side with me when I concocted a story about arriving at the hospital feeling unwell and the doctor deciding to keep me in for investigation.

Now I'm back at school, attending weekly sessions of therapy. My teaching is fine but my private life is fraught with loneliness and self-loathing.

*

Doctor Lessier, my psychiatrist, leans back in his chair calmly puffing on his pipe, watching me light a cigarette.

"Please tell me what to *do*. My life is all

messed up."

"You're looking for the Big Breast again," he sighs. He's often said that in the three months I've been seeing him.

I'm confused. I don't know what he's trying to imply.

"I don't know what you *mean*," I say angrily.

He doesn't answer me. My anger turns to hopelessness.

"*Please* put me in the hospital."

"No – I won't do that." He looks at his watch. "Time's up. See you next week."

"You *won't* see me – I'm not coming again."

He shrugs and opens the door.

I leave feeling as desperate as when I arrived.

During the past few weeks at school the despair has become overwhelming. Every time I see the Principal's kind, calm face I long for her to hold me close, talk to me gently, promise me that she will look after me always. My mind knows I must not regard her as a mother figure. At twenty-three years old I'm a teacher, not a small, helpless child. But the little girl inside me doesn't understand. She won't accept the adult concept. She's still looking for a warm, loving mummy to care for her every need, a mummy she cannot have because this woman is a nun, her life devoted to God, the Catholic Church and the school.

Now she's really worried about me. I'm getting no better. Sometimes I have to leave the classroom early to go home because it's becoming increasingly difficult to contain my emotions.

I ring her on leaving the doctor's office.

"I'm going to admit myself to the mental hospital on the hill." I can't hold back the tears as I talk.

"If you do that I shall have no option but to tell the School Board." Her voice is quiet, sympathetic as she continues, "I shall send a priest to your house to take you. Are you quite sure you want to go?"

"Yes – I've got to," I reply.

The priest arrives soon after I return home. He doesn't try to engage me in conversation except to ask, "Are you certain you want to do this? You can change your mind, it's not too late."

"If I don't go into hospital I won't be able to cope."

He drives me the short distance up what is known locally as The Mountain. The Reception staff do not want to admit me.

"If you don't I'll take my life."

I leave them with no alternative. The priest leaves. I'm taken to a small ward with several beds, all empty. The nurse gives me some tablets. She doesn't explain what they're for. She waits until I've taken them.

"This is your bed," she says matter-of-factly, pointing out the one nearest the door. She turns, walks away without so much as a backward glance.

I feel terribly unhappy. I don't want to stay here. I lie down feeling so alone, so mixed up…

*

I'm woken by a nurse. I see her through a haze. I feel like I've had far too much to drink.

"Get up. I'm taking you to another ward," she says gruffly.

I struggle off the bed. It's an enormous effort. My mind feels sluggish. I can't think clearly. My body doesn't want to move. I feel faint standing up. I hold onto the rail at the end of the bed. "I don't think I can go anywhere," I mumble.

"Hurry up! I haven't got all day," she snaps.

Reluctantly I follow her.

She opens the door, waits for me to go through and locks it behind me. A long corridor with chairs down one side stretches before me.

She takes the bag I've brought with me, packed with clothes and toiletries.

"You won't need this at the moment," she says briskly. "We need to label everything."

A doctor comes to examine me.

"How long do you think it will be before you lose your job?" he asks.

"They won't sack me – I'm a good teacher," I reply.

He smiles at the nurse beside him. I'm puzzled. I don't understand what he's implying.

Later that morning I sit with other women in the corridor. We're each allowed to keep a packet of cigarettes but only one match an hour is provided so we chain-smoke our way through the long day.

There's an ancient piano in the dining room but after playing a few notes I lose interest.

A psychologist breaks the monotony by doing a battery of psychological tests with me. For a short while I enjoy the mental stimulation, forgetting where I am.

Apart from the Principal, who visits briefly with a present of a pair of slippers, I see nobody I know. I'm frustrated, angry. I can't even escape into sleep as we're not permitted to lie down during the day. There are no doors on the toilets or the bathrooms; no privacy, no humanity. Endless, empty time...

I've had enough. I walk decisively to the heavy wooden door at the end of the corridor. I know exactly what I'm going to do. I bang hard with both fists.

"Let me out!" I keep shouting until nurses come running.

"If you carry on like this you'll be locked up," one of them says coldly. "Go and sit in the corridor with the others."

But I'm past caring. I hate it here. I want to go.

I continue beating the door with all my energy. My arms are pulled behind my back. I'm frog-marched down to the washroom area. A door is flung open. I'm being pushed into a narrow cell with green brick walls and high, closed windows. I'm stripped of my clothes, left standing on the cold stone floor. Apart from a mattress in one corner the room is empty.

I hear a loud slam and the sound of a key turning in the lock. There's no way out.

The grille in the wooden door is opened. A hostile face glares at me.

"Please don't leave me here like this," I beg.

"You will stay in there until you cool down," the stern voice commands. There is no kindness in those eyes.

I have nothing to cover myself. I crouch in a corner of the room, my arms wrapped tightly round my body in a vain attempt to conceal my nakedness.

Women passing on their way to the toilet peer curiously at this freak. I cower further against the hard wall frantically wishing I could disappear into it. I'm a wounded animal, panicking, trapped, sick with fear.

"I must get out before I wet myself!" I plead with the next nurse to stare through the grille.

I hear the clank of keys.

"Promise not to bang on the door again?" the nurse asks, glowering at me.

There's no choice. If I'm to be released I'll have to do anything they ask. There's no fight left in me.

A nurse hands me my clothes. I dress hurriedly, afraid she might change her mind, lock me up again.

She hands me my coat.

"Put this on," she says without explanation.

I stare at it disbelieving, horrified. My name has been scribbled in huge letters with black pen across the lining of my prized, brand-new camelhair coat.

As I'm herded in a group through the hospital grounds for the daily short walk I can think of nothing but the cruel damage to the coat I was so proud of.

I've lost everything – my freedom, my dignity, my mind. And it's *my* fault. I demanded to be in this prison.

*

Every night I wake drenched in sweat from dreams replaying my distress. Each time they end with my Principal rescuing me, showing me how to live my life differently.

I keep trying to work out how I can get back to Canada to be with her again. Each day is filled with torturous thoughts.

Over and over I keep thinking I should never have incarcerated myself in that mental hospital. It doesn't take much intelligence to realise that declaring myself suicidal would inevitably result in the loss of the new life I was trying to make for myself in Canada. Who in their right mind would continue to employ me as a teacher, however competent I'd shown myself to be? If it hadn't been for a friend of the family who had emigrated to Toronto, I don't know what would have happened to me.

My last clear memory is of the Director of the School Board saying, "We'll pay you until the summer in lieu of the usual three months' notice."

I unashamedly begged him to let me return, give me another chance to prove my emotional stability in the classroom. "You know I'm a good teacher…"

"The decision is final," he said from behind his glasses, behind his desk, a clear warning in his eyes to argue no further against my dismissal.

I phoned Mummy's friend. She packed my trunk, sold my television, gave me papers to sign authorising withdrawal of money from the bank, used the money to buy flowers for my Principal and to buy me an air ticket. She sorted my clothes out for the journey, placed me in the care of an air hostess.

Those last days in Canada were a waking nightmare, any element of control, any ability to make the simplest decision gone. Drugs ensured I slept most of the flight.

*

For the next three months I lived in a drugged, twilight world, afraid to leave the house, unable to talk to anyone. Most days I didn't bother to get washed or dressed, just sat in a chair gazing into space. I scarcely noticed anything that happened. Occasionally, the doctor visited with a prescription for more tranquillizers. All I wanted to do was sleep, to blot out the pain of being the failure that I felt I'd become.

Even Mummy, unusually for her, left me to my own devices. I had no idea why she no longer nagged me incessantly or railed about my selfishness and neither did I care. Nothing, nobody was important, not even Mummy.

Daddy tried to motivate me; "Do something today, anything," he would urge before leaving for work. "Don't just sit in that chair. Go into the garden, throw a ball to the dog."

Mummy showed me an advertisement for a job.

'Nanny wanted for two small children in Paris.'

I wrote, not expecting a reply. Within a month

I was boarding the plane for France.

I was the fourth nanny in two years. Before long I understood why. It was prestigious to employ an English nanny. But I was not prepared to be a mother substitute for two little girls who were desperate for a share of their Mummy's attention. I knew only too well how that felt.

I had been there barely two weeks when two-year-old Olivia woke screaming from a nightmare. Unable to comfort her I asked her mother to console her. She responded by telling me to spank the child if she continued to cry. My refusal angered her.

After six months my French had improved. I had a job lined up in Gibraltar to teach children of Royal Navy and R.A.F. families and anger had fuelled my mental recovery. When I was sacked for refusing to take the children for a walk in the rain I was able to cope.

*

Gibraltar was an experience with a difference. I was happy to be teaching once again and relieved that the Ministry of Defence had not tried to get a reference from the school board in Canada.

Eventually I tired of cocktail parties on board visiting warships and evenings out with married officers. Dennis, who taught at the same school as I did, was single, kind-hearted, warm and loving with a fantastic sense of humour. And when after a year he asked me to marry him, I knew I was lucky to have found someone who was willing to put up with the emotionally unstable person I felt I was. The final seal was put on our future when Mummy met and approved of the man I had chosen to spend my life with.

Chapter Three

We've just returned from three years in Gibraltar and we're staying with Mummy. In a couple of weeks we're leaving for Iran to teach at an international school. We're excited at the prospect. The downside is the batch of vaccinations we've had to endure before we go.

Dennis and I have both woken up feeling terribly ill. We were warned that yesterday's jab could have unpleasant after-effects but we weren't prepared for a reaction of this sort. Unable to get out of bed we compare symptoms. They're the same: aching joints and muscles, excruciating headache, feverishness... It's like we've developed the worst case of 'flu.

Normally we'd stay in bed, wait till the symptoms eased. But we're at Mummy's house and she doesn't take kindly to anyone remaining in bed after nine a.m. at the latest. It's ten o'clock already.

I can hear loud footsteps coming upstairs.

The door bursts open.

"Aren't you up yet? I had breakfast ready over an hour ago," Mummy grumbles. The way she's looking at us is akin to disgust. I sense that she doesn't approve of us sharing a bed, despite being married. She and Daddy have had single beds for many years. Before that a bolster divided their double bed.

"We can't get up. We're feeling awful. It was that injection yesterday," I say, knowing that my weak protests will make no difference.

"Don't be ridiculous! Everyone going abroad has those and *they* don't make a fuss. There's nothing wrong with you. Just get up and forget about it."

She strides out of the room. She neither waits for nor expects a reply.

Dennis hasn't seen this side of Mummy.

"I suppose we'd better get up," he says, struggling to his feet. He gets dressed.

I can't even manage that. I put on my dressing gown. It's an effort. The mere act of standing is causing my head to swim.

We drag ourselves downstairs. Neither of us can eat the breakfast Mummy has prepared.

"Do you know, you're really ungrateful!" She stands, hands on hips, watching our feeble attempts to eat.

I can see by Dennis' face he's feeling sick too.

But Mummy's not about to give up.

"All this nonsense over one tiny injection! I have to have them monthly for my anaemia. When do you ever hear *me* complain?"

She storms off into the kitchen.

"I'm not putting up with this!" Dennis snaps suddenly. "I can't listen to any more. I'm going out."

His face is white. How's he going to cope? Mummy might treat *me* like this, but why is she so unfeeling towards Dennis? What has he ever done to deserve it?

I can see how difficult it is for him to put his coat on. I wish I could go with him but I wouldn't get halfway down the road.

I hear the front door close behind him. I rest my head on the table, cry bitter, resentful, noiseless tears for him, for me, for the lack of a Mummy who cares...

*

After a few months in Iran we wanted desperately to return to England. I had got used to huge cockroaches and the sweltering heat. We had a good social life and I had established a successful international choir in our school. But there were iron bars on windows and a constant fear of the secret police, present at every public function; one word against the Shah spelt instant imprisonment. Our life of comparative luxury compared with the extreme poverty among local people meant either turning a blind eye to their daily plight or getting out of the country since we were powerless to change their lives. The final straw was the death of a ten-year-old in Dennis' class who was left to die on a lonely, unlit road after a hit-and-run accident.

My becoming pregnant provided an excuse to break our two-year contract.

But once back in England, with Dennis unemployed and me nursing my mother-in-law, who was dying of cancer, I became deeply depressed. The only help I was offered during my pregnancy was a low dose of Valium.

When Simon was born I tried to ignore my low physical and mental state. Dennis had another teaching post and we bought a little terraced house in a small market town in Suffolk. I took up supply teaching and we had another baby, a beautiful little girl whom we called Rachel. To any outsider we were a normal, happy family.

*

I should be content with my life. I have two wonderful children, I'm pregnant with my third, have a loyal husband and a comfortable home.

But there seems to be no end to my deep depression, my intense dislike of myself.

I've been attending weekly sessions for the past four years with Katherine, a psychotherapist. I can hardly wait to see her each week. Either she comes to my house or the hospital sends transport for me.

Today I'm at the hospital. Katherine listens attentively, gives sympathetic responses and seems to understand my frustrated attempts to please Mummy, to get her to love me. But although I spend the hour talking practically non-stop about my problems I'm no closer to finding answers to them.

And worryingly, I've become extremely dependent on Katherine. She's the kind of person I long to be mothered by, caring, kind and compassionate. Her intelligent brown eyes and gentle voice acknowledge my emotional pain. And she never makes fun of me if I cry but encourages me to talk freely, openly, about my feelings. She understands my distress at discovering, during an argument with another seven-year-old in the playground, that I was adopted, at finding out that other children and their parents knew I was different. Unlike Mummy, she doesn't attribute my feelings to an over-active imagination. She accepts them as normal reactions to my upbringing.

I feel guilty whenever I talk about my adoptive parents. I find excuses for the frequent beatings from Daddy that left me bleeding and bruised. I try to justify Mummy's attacks on me, the daily scorn she poured on everything I did, her contempt for the way I failed to match up to her own daughter, her disgust at the person I was and still am. But Katherine quietly urges me to explore each situation further.

She listens patiently as I tell her about my fear of going to hell when I die, if I commit a mortal sin like missing Mass on a Sunday, my frustration at my inability to be perfect like the saints the nuns at my Catholic school told me about. She looks concerned when I tell her how traumatic it was attending a ten-year-old classmate's funeral and our teacher saying afterwards: "Evelyn's gone to Heaven because she was a good girl, but what if it had been one of you...?"

I can express any opinion and she accepts that this is how I feel. The more I get to know her, the greater my warmth and respect for her.

I suspect she cares a lot about me. On one occasion she accepted an invitation to our house warming and she came to visit me in the maternity ward when Rachel was born. Things Mummy's never done.

She lives with her grown-up daughter. I know she's split with her husband. He was a Catholic. The divorce was messy, left her feeling hurt and resentful. She's talked to me briefly about it.

During this session she's mentioned her daughter several times. I gather from her comments that there's a strong bond between them. I fantasise about her daughter and me getting on well together.

On impulse, I ask timidly, "Could you think of *me* as part of your family?" I can't help sounding like a small child.

She recoils visibly. I've taken her off-guard. She throws me a look resembling disgust.

"Of course not!" She leans back in her chair, obviously tense, silent, shocked by what I've asked.

She might as well have slapped my face. I can't handle this. If she doesn't want me as a daughter I don't want to see her again. The one way forward, as I see it, would have been for her to mother me, give me what I didn't have. But she hasn't the slightest intention of complying with my request or coming to some sort of compromise.

"Well I don't want to see you again!" I exclaim petulantly.

"Perhaps we could meet less often – say once a fortnight, " she suggests.

"No – you don't care enough about me. I'm going – and I'm never coming back." I know the hurt shows on my face.

"It's not wise but it has to be your decision," she says quietly.

Walking out of the room I half expect her to call me back, change her mind, agree to be a surrogate mother for me.

But she closes the door behind me. I feel like I did during the times Mummy locked me out of the house when I was a child. I want to return, beg her to reconsider…

But I know it's too late. I've ruined our therapeutic relationship. She's not going to see me again.

*

I put my past on the back burner, tried to avoid looking in the mirror at what appeared to be a very ugly reflection and concentrated on the problems I was having with the new baby. From the time he began to crawl Nathan seemed to bruise easily. When I took him in his pram to collect Simon and Rachel from school, other parents would avoid talking to me, give me accusing looks. With nasty-looking purple, raised shiny bruises on his forehead, arms and legs he did look like a victim of child battering.

Refusing to be brushed off by our G.P.'s comment, "Some children do bruise easily," I made frequent visits to the surgery in an attempt to find out what was wrong with Nathan. Deep down I suspected that it was something serious. But each time I was branded as a fussy mother.

When Nathan was twenty-one months old a diagnosis of severe haemophilia sent me into a state of inner panic. Doctors appeared to know little about the condition and I feared for our tiny son who suddenly seemed terribly fragile. Whilst I became extremely over-protective Dennis coped better, taking Nathan for long walks to strengthen his leg muscles and giving me a chance to rest – I was six months pregnant. We could not, however, discuss our shared trauma, which added to the emotional burden that I felt increasingly unable to cope with.

*

A recent scan showed that I'm probably carrying a girl, which means that this baby won't be affected like Nathan.

This day in the labour room is the first respite we've had since the diagnosis three months ago. We read books, listen to music and relax. But in the evening doctors decide to speed up my well-spaced contractions. A short while later I feel a strong urge to push...

"It's a little boy," the midwife says quietly. She knows why I desperately wanted a girl.

Every part of me hurts. She must have got it wrong. This can't be happening.

Dennis is cradling our baby son. I bury my face in the pillow.

"Look at him, darling, he's beautiful," Dennis says.

I turn my head slowly. Dennis leans forward to kiss me, bringing the tiny body in a white blanket close to my face.

A searing pain shoots through me. An overwhelming tide of emotion sweeps through my body. I feel utterly helpless, completely unable to prevent its release. All the unexpressed emotion about Nathan's haemophilia is flooding out of me in a seemingly unending rush.

I can hear a primitive, piercing sound like the wailing of an animal in extreme pain. I'm dimly aware that it's coming from me but can do nothing to control it. It takes two tranquillising injections to calm me.

I breast-feed Benjamin, but I feel nothing...

*

No counselling was offered as, back home, I struggled with postnatal depression, knowing I would have to wait until my baby was six months old before being sure that he did not have haemophilia. Tests were unreliable just after birth.

I lived in a drugged, apathetic world, only vaguely aware of what was happening around me. I fed my baby whenever he cried but did little else.

Sometimes a small curly head nuzzled against my arm, a soft hand gently stroked my cheek.

"Mummy tired," Nathan would say.

*

It's nighttime. All four children are sleeping and Dennis is listening to music through his headphones downstairs. Nothing is going to change; I shall never be able to get Dennis to discuss emotional issues that affect us both. Benjamin has probably got haemophilia and I won't be able to cope. I shall always be the stupid, useless person Mummy told me I was. I don't deserve the beautiful children I have. I must find a way out.

I swallow a few handfuls of sleeping tablets.

Almost immediately I regret what I've done. All I can think of is that I mustn't abandon my baby.

I pick up the phone, dial 999.

"I've taken an overdose."

"We'll send an ambulance."

"No, wait, I'm only coming in if I can bring my baby with me."

There's a pause.

"How old is the baby?"

"Eight weeks."

"We'll take you both."

I walk unsteadily downstairs to tell Dennis what I've done. My words are slurred. The room is spinning…

*

After nearly three weeks in the Mother & Baby Unit, staying in my room with Benjamin, constantly fearing that another patient in the psychiatric wing might harm or abduct him, I persuaded the doctor to allow us to go home. We had saved hard for a year, having finally traced my birth mother, to fly to the U.S.A. to meet her for the first time. The flight was booked, the children were looking forward to meeting their nana and I had high hopes of finding someone who would be able to give me the love I'd so desperately craved from my adoptive parents.

But the experience wasn't the fairy-tale ending I'd dreamed about. My mother, racked with feelings of guilt, inadequacy and loss, had long ago given up on herself. Crippled with arthritis and housebound, she'd lost all interest in herself. The grossly-overweight woman propped up on crutches, her mouth sagging without the support of her false teeth, her greying hair unkempt, wearing no make up, was a far cry from the photograph I carried of a smiling lady with sleek, glossy hair framing an attractive face. And although she had never stopped loving me and was delighted to see me, she constantly told me how giving me up had ruined her life. Seeing the lack of respect with which my half-brother treated her and watching her husband, who had schizophrenia, I could only feel terribly sorry and somehow responsible for her unhappy life. I knew then I could never express the anger I felt about being given up for adoption. To do that would have been heartless and cruel.

Chapter Four

"That's the third bottle of vodka you've got through this week. I bet you couldn't go without a drink for the next three days."

Dennis' challenge hits home like a stone. And inwardly I am forced to face the unpleasant truth that he's right. I haven't given a thought to the amount I've been drinking. Until he said that, I was blissfully ignorant of the fact that I've slipped quite far down the slope towards alcoholism.

I'm consumed with anger at Mummy's silence. She hasn't spoken to me for over a year, ever since I phoned to tell her I'd found my natural mother. I can't tolerate the rift. I feel abandoned, rejected. As if I needed further proof that I'm worth nothing, Teresa informed me that Mummy has cut me out of her will.

I *won't* have another glass of alcohol tonight. I'll prove to Dennis that I'm not an alcoholic. If *he* rejects me I'll have no one. But I can't resist the urge to vent my horrendous rage.

I wait until 11.30: Mummy goes to bed early. My heart is beating incredibly fast as I walk up the road to the phone box. My finger trembles as I dial her number. I wait. I picture her getting out of bed, putting on her slippers, coming down the stairs extremely annoyed, wondering who can be ringing yet again this late at night. I smile, imagining her face.

"Who is it?" A brief pause… "I'm sick and tired of this!"

I listen to her irritation with grim satisfaction, visualising her impatience as she waits for a reply. She's not used to her demands being responded to with nothing more than the sound of breathing.

I hold on for a few seconds longer, my stomach churning. It's stifling in here. I replace the receiver, move out into the freshness of the night.

*

Last year was horrible. Daddy died in August after several years suffering from Alzheimer's disease. I'd been shocked at the dramatic change in him when Mummy brought him to the Christening of Joel, our fifth child. She had finally relented after nearly two years without speaking to me, responded to the invitation we'd sent. I'd always known Daddy loved me in spite of the terrible beatings. And I had loved him intensely. It was acutely painful watching him deteriorate month by month, until he sat blank-faced in the corner of a bleak psychiatric ward for the elderly, in Shenley – the hospital I'd stayed in overnight at the age of twenty-one. My Daddy, the last time I saw him, after a brief moment of recognition, had lapsed into a place where nobody could reach him.

It was a conscious decision on our part to have another child whom we hoped would, like Ben, be unaffected by haemophilia. But bringing up five children wasn't easy. And Dennis, although enjoying reading bedtime stories to them, was reluctant to make rules. I was the one who timetabled their day and set the behaviour limits.

And in so doing I felt like the bad parent.

I learned to give Nathan the injections of his missing blood-clotting factor to avoid wasted hours going to hospital but it took months before I was able to get the needle into his vein at the first attempt. And inflicting pain on my young son felt unbearable.

With Dennis' new appointment as deputy head we moved north. The children seemed to settle quickly and I finished my book about Haemophilia. But Mummy wasn't impressed when my sister gave her a copy. Her scornful comments cut through me. If Mummy didn't value my writing then it couldn't possibly be worthwhile.

In the same year my natural mother died of lung cancer, caused by years of heavy smoking. I flew out with two-year-old Joel, the grandchild she had never seen, was at her bedside when she drifted gently away from me just when we were beginning to form a closer bond. And she valued what I did.

"My daughter has written a book," she announced proudly to the doctor when he visited. Her death felt like she had abandoned me all over again. I felt alone, empty, afraid…

This year hasn't started much better. I've had an operation to remove loose bodies floating round my kneecap. I can hardly walk, let alone manage the running of a home and children…

And the anti-depressants and painkillers aren't working. Following a home visit from a psychiatrist who spent some time trying to persuade me to go into hospital, I'm waiting for transport for an appointment with him. The older children are at school but Joel comes everywhere with me.

The car is on time. We're both ready. There's no one else to pick up so the journey takes just fifteen minutes.

A nurse looks after Joel while Doctor Kay takes me to his office. He fetches a chair from behind his desk, places it close to mine.

"You're still very depressed," he says simply.

"I'm not quite so bad." I'm trying to show I'm making an effort.

"I haven't changed my mind. You still need to be admitted to the ward. I want you to come in today."

This is too sudden for me. "I can't!" I protest. "I've got Joel with me and there's nobody to look after him."

"I can ring your husband. I'm sure we can sort something out between us. If you'll agree to stay I'll make sure you get physiotherapy for your knee, too." His brown eyes are full of concern. He really cares about me.

I can feel myself weakening. He's strong, I'm not. He's leaning towards me, urging me to reconsider, offering me relief from this nightmare of mental suffering, immediate treatment for my painful knee.

"I'm not sure what to do." I can hear my voice faltering.

"Let us help you." The warmth of his tone is overwhelming. I begin to cry softly.

"It won't be for long," he adds gently.

I have no will left. The doctor's voice is hypnotic. I'm compelled to agree, my last bit of resistance used up.

"If you think it will be good for me," I say in a weak voice.

Without a moment's hesitation he picks up the phone. From what he's saying, I know he's speaking to Dennis.

"Right. It's all arranged," he says briskly. "Come with me."

He's taken over. I'm not responsible for myself any more. As if in a dream, I walk past Joel and the nurse playing with brightly coloured toys, along numerous corridors to another wing of the hospital.

I'm filled with fear, yet I'm clinging to the doctor's promise of my mental and physical recovery.

We go through double doors into a ward where Doctor Kay speaks briefly to a nurse, smiles at me and leaves.

I watch his departing back. I feel lost without him.

"Come with me," the nurse says, not unkindly.

I'm escorted to a small room.

"Right. I need some details from you…"

The paperwork finished, she takes me to a large room, brings me a cup of tea. Sipping it slowly, I take a look around me.

There's a game show on the television but no one's watching it. A shabbily dressed middle-aged man is shuffling about the room. He's chanting from a book, oblivious to anyone around him. A teenage girl is slumped in an armchair, gazing vacantly out of the window. An old woman, stockings halfway down her legs, is snoring in a corner. They're all closeted in a world of their own.

The nurse takes me to a room with curtained cubicles. A bed and small chest of drawers fill the entire space. Several other patients are sleeping, their curtains wide open. I cry quietly so as not to disturb them. As always, I'm terrified of making someone angry with me.

My face is still wet with tears when Dennis arrives. He looks so sad.

"Please take me home. I can't stay here," I beg him.

"Well... we need to talk to someone before I can do that," he replies.

For the next hour the nurse listens to my reasons for wanting to leave. I talk round and round in circles.

"Just give it one night. See how you feel then. You're a voluntary patient. If you still want to leave in the morning, you'll be free to go. It's getting late now."

Reluctantly I agree, on the condition that I'm given a room to myself. I'm frightened that the man pacing the corridor, shouting at people passing, will attack me. The nurse complies with my request.

In spite of the sleeping tablets and the closed door I'm shaking, afraid of the man, wondering how safe I am here.

I wake frequently, soaked in sweat from my nightmares.

I resolve to get out of this place first thing in the morning.

*

I get up late, too late for breakfast. Washing my face in the sink in the corner, I notice the water goes down the plughole and forms a pool on the floor below. I mention it to someone at the nursing station. She doesn't look up from her newspaper, just nods her acknowledgement.

That's it, I decide; if I remain here I'll go completely mad like the rest of them.

Quickly I pack the few belongings Dennis brought in for me, search for a different nurse. The staff don't wear uniforms here but I come across a pleasant-looking man whose badge says simply, "Liam – Charge Nurse."

"I want to go home. I've cried a lot and I'm sure I'll be able to cope now."

"How will you get back?" he asks.

"I've got enough money for a taxi," I assure him.

"Right. Well, your son is being looked after in the crèche down the hallway. Your husband brought him in this morning while you were asleep. I'll have to inform Doctor Kay that you want to go."

"That's fine." I say, relieved that it's all so easy. I can hardly wait to taste freedom. It was a mistake coming here, I know that now.

Doctor Kay arrives within minutes of being contacted. "I'll deal with this," he informs Liam.

There's a sign on the door of the room he takes me into. It says Quiet Room. I sit on a chair close to the door while the doctor selects one on the far side of the room.

"What's this I hear about you wanting to go home?" he demands. Gone is the soft, seducing tone of the day before, the concerned body language. His words are clipped, he's leaning back in his chair, arms folded across his chest.

Taken totally by surprise at his change of attitude, I stare wordlessly at him, unable to speak.

"You're not leaving today and that's final." He says it in a way not to be argued with, rather like Mummy when as a child I asked if I could go to a friend's house to play.

"But I'm a voluntary patient! You can't keep me here against my will. I haven't threatened to harm myself or anyone else."

"I can do what I like." His voice is slow, the tone menacing. "I can detain you for thirty-six hours without consulting anyone."

I'm trapped, stunned into silence. Surely he can't do this – can he?

Without waiting for a reply, he strides from the room. I follow him. I hear him say loudly, "If she tries to leave – stop her."

And he's gone. I'm in a prison. I can't get out.

"He can't do that!" My head's in a whirl. "I came in as a voluntary patient," I protest to Liam.

"Yes – I think it's wrong too. I'll see what can be done about it."

The whole thing's getting worse; I'm now being humoured to prevent me making a sudden bolt for the door.

Deflated, I sink onto a chair, wondering how

I'm going to deal with yet another mess I've got myself into...

I don't know how long I've been sitting here dazed, unable to think clearly, when Liam interrupts my thoughts.

"Right. I agree with you. You shouldn't be forced to stay here but I'm in a difficult position. All I'll say is that Doctor Kay's in a meeting till 12.30. If you can get your husband to collect you before then, I know nothing about it. Obviously at some point we'll have to let the doctor know you've left."

He means it! He really is on my side!

I've got to act fast if I'm to get out. What if Doctor Kay's meeting finishes early and he holds Joel captive so I can't leave?

I dial Dennis' school number, explain the situation. "We haven't got long," I say urgently.

Half an hour later he's at the door. "I've left the car round the other side of the building," he tells me. "You go straight there. I'll collect Joel."

It's a race against time.

"I'm going now," I tell Liam. "Please give me long enough to get clear of here... and thank you," I call over my shoulder.

I spend the afternoon at a safe house belonging to a friend of a friend. I daren't go home. Even though no one knows where I am, I spend the afternoon dreading a knock on the door. Cowering in a chair in a corner of the conservatory, I'm convinced that Doctor Kay, furious at my departure, will arrive at any moment with police in tow and force me to return to the ward.

His betrayal of trust reminds me of another instance in my life when our family doctor, a man I respected, let me down, left me feeling disgusted with myself and frightened like I do now. I was thirteen years old when, just before opening the surgery door to show me out, he leaned down and kissed me full on the mouth. I shudder at the memory of the taste of his breath.

Back home, I relax slightly. I'm with Dennis and the children and so far there's been no dreaded appearance of the doctor.

But I daren't go outside the house, just in case...

*

I telephoned a counsellor for MIND, a national mental health organisation, that evening. Their advisor agreed that in trying to detain me when I had been admitted on a voluntary basis, the doctor was out of order in using his sectioning power, especially as I had given no cause for further concern. I was reassured that although he could still attempt to admit me forcibly it would now require two people to visit, assess me and decide that I was sectionable.

I waited anxiously over the next few days. Nobody came to even check if I was alive. There was no follow-up letter. I began to feel extremely angry. I wrote to the Health Authority complaining about what had happened. Following a full investigation they expressed "grave concerns" about the doctor's treatment of me, which they had voiced to him and they now left the ball in his court and hoped that a satisfactory outcome would ensue.

Doctor Kay wrote to me but his letter, far from being an apology, stated that he would be prepared to take the same action given a repeat performance of the circumstances. I felt dismissed, unimportant and depressed. It seemed I was simply not worth the suggested apology.

Eventually, I plucked up the courage to visit my G. P. who said she would try to get therapy for me but warned it could take some time. Meanwhile, I tried to ignore the way I felt and threw myself into supply teaching and coping with the demands of family life. The sensations of emptiness, isolation and self-hatred did not diminish. In fact, the more I suppressed them the unhappier I became. Late at night I would often frantically change the entire contents of a room around – an obsessive habit, which the children found exciting, enjoying the new arrangement that greeted them in the morning, but which Dennis found annoying and unsettling. However, rather than tell me how he felt, he withdrew to his study preferring to ignore the upheaval that was taking place on an almost daily basis.

Chapter Five

Agitation, confusion, fear, are escalating within me as I follow the psychotherapist into the large, comfortable, airy sitting-room where we've met each week for the past month. This room seems strangely at odds with the torture of the therapy.

I've been on a waiting list for two years, growing increasingly desperate. I felt such relief when I was finally assessed and accepted for this place. At last, I thought, I'm on the right track to understanding and learning how to deal with my problems. I've found someone to guide me through the maze, help me to cope with life in a positive, constructive manner…

And then I was introduced to Nadia.

Initially things looked hopeful. She asked me about myself and what sort of therapies I'd had before. That took up the first ten minutes of the session. And then she seemed to dry up. She relaxed back into the chair opposite me and said nothing. Of course I waited for more questions, perhaps some direction…

But the silence continued, became difficult, uncomfortable.

The next three sessions were the same; apart from the initial greeting Nadia simply sat and watched me, her face totally impassive.

Nervously, I talked randomly about various childhood incidents, overdoses, in fact anything that came into my head.

Occasionally she'd make a comment such as,

"Mmm… that seems to leave you feeling frustrated / lonely / sad…" or whatever seemed appropriate at the time.

But I knew that anyway. It was quite obvious even to me, from the way I spoke about things, what my feelings were. I'm not *that* stupid.

Today I'm getting more and more irritable. "What do you want me to talk about?"

Nadia smiles but says nothing.

"It's not funny! I don't know what I'm supposed to be doing. It's not helping me rambling on about this and that…"

"You're angry," she states calmly. Her expression seems smug, superior. I'm being humiliated.

"Of course I'm angry! I don't need a psychologist to tell me *that*!"

She doesn't respond. How *dare* she sit there, letting me talk round in circles, wind myself up further and further into a frantic frenzy.

"You get paid for sitting there doing nothing," I accuse her. "Just telling me things I already know!"

Still she doesn't react; not a flicker of emotion.

I watch the clock, resolve to spend the remaining time in silence, if that's what she wants. I pass ten minutes studying pictures on the walls. Nadia's eyes remain firmly fixed on my face.

The discomfort becomes too great. I'm feeling too self-conscious.

I begin to waffle about the style of the artist who created the paintings around us. It's all I can think of to talk about.

She's still watching me.

Suddenly I burst out in exasperation, "What a waste of time this is! And *I* don't even get paid for it." I can't think of anything else to say. It's like talking to a robot – she's not really human. If she were she'd see how lost, how helpless, how hopeless I feel.

I avoid looking at her, try to pretend she's not here. I plan how I'd arrange this room if it were in my house.

"That's it!" Her voice startles me back to reality.

"I'll see you next week," I say lamely.

"No you won't. I'm not seeing you any more."

The finality of her dismissal hits me like a stone.

"You can't *do* that! I know it's not working but I'm willing to come each week to see if I can get *some*where. You can't give up on me like this."

"It's over," she says firmly, decisively. I can see she's not going to change her mind. She doesn't think I'm sufficiently important to merit treatment.

"Well, sod you!" I exclaim, glaring directly into her eyes.

I turn, walk away fast. For a second I'm tempted to rush back, apologise, plead with her to forgive me, give me another chance. But I know it would be pointless. She's clearly written me off.

*

It's Saturday morning. I've woken early, unable to get the face of the nun, the Headmistress of my current school, out of my head.

I know my dependency on her is futile. I'm aware I see her as a replacement for Mummy. And I realise I'm trapped in my agonising longing for her warmth. The Child inside me is crying out for her attention; the lack of it is destroying me.

Inspectors, parents, children respond so positively to my teaching but the Head of our school remains unmoved by my enthusiasm, my skills as a teacher. And hers is the sole approval I crave. I cannot give it to myself. It means little from others.

If I don't deserve her praise for my efforts in the classroom I must find another way to make her care for me.

The adult part of me knows The Child is desperate. Today the Little Girl is screaming for Mummy. I'm fighting not to let her take me over. I'm losing. She can't bear being ignored.

I'm so confused. I can't get out of bed. A horrible thought is developing in my head, returning with increasing strength whenever I dismiss it. I can think of no other way to make Sister notice me, make me feel special to her.

My heart is beating fast. I've played this game twice before in my life. Will it work again?
Something is urging me strongly, daring me to try.

I can't resist it. I remain in bed, staring out of the window at the rooftops, knowing that at any point I can decide not to go through with it, get up, carry on as normal.
I struggle out of bed, go downstairs, drink several glasses of water, return to bed.

Hours pass...

I hate the waiting, the feeling of needing to use the toilet, forbidding myself to go, becoming more and more uncomfortable. I'm arguing with myself to break this cycle of destruction. The Child is convinced that Mummy, in the shape of Sister, will feel sorry for her if I have to go into hospital.

It's early evening. The cramping tension in my lower abdomen is so intense I have to act. I can't think clearly. Pain is blocking everything out.

I tell Dennis I'm unable to pass water. The doctor visits, calls an ambulance. Things happen quickly. I'm catheterised, given a pain-killing injection that makes my surroundings look fuzzy.

Suddenly Sister is there in the ward, sitting beside me, talking to me kindly.

"I knew you weren't well this week," she says softly.

I'm melting inside. The Child is rewarded. She feels loved. She's got what she wanted – for now...

Sister is leaving. It's been a short visit. I want to scream, "Please come back! Take me home with you! Look after me, I don't need to be in hospital, there's nothing wrong with my body, I just need to be with you, to be loved by you..."

But I silence The Child, say nothing. And as Sister walks away I'm left with a tremendous sense of shame and an overwhelming feeling of loss.

*

I've just finished another day's teaching in the

school where I have a good rapport with the children, run a successful choir and continue to be highly praised by everyone except the Headmistress. When she isn't avoiding me she's criticising anything I say or do. I'll never be able to please her however hard I try. And without her approval I am nothing, nobody.

My classroom is quiet now that the children and the other teachers have gone home. I'm sitting staring out of the window, seeing nothing. Sister is in her office downstairs, working late to deal with paperwork. Perhaps I should go to her, tell her how unhappy I am, how hurt that nothing I do is good enough for her. How stupid! I think angrily. Do I really expect her to listen to me as though I am a little girl, to reassure me with a hug and kind words?

I feel very desperate. I must do something. There has to a way to make myself feel better. But Mummy thinks I'm useless and Sister isn't interested in me. Dennis is wrapped up in his professional life and coping with our children as well as fulltime teaching is too much for me. I feel lost, lonely and, worst of all, I can't stand the self-pity. I can't think of anything I can do to take away the self-hatred, the mounting desperation, the overwhelming emotional pain. And it's not going to stop…

Suddenly I think of the painkillers and tranquillizers in my bag. They might not solve my problems but, if I take enough, they will blank out this awful vice-like grip round my head, they'll put an end to the screaming inside…

My hands are trembling, it's difficult to undo the child-proof bottle caps. But now I've decided what to do there's no going back. It's like I'm compelled to finish what I started without knowing why. And the reason doesn't matter any more.

Everything in the room is hazy. I feel very relaxed. No worries, no problems, no feelings…

I'm thirsty. I'll go and make myself a coffee. I hold onto the stair rail, the stairs seem to be moving as I stagger down them…

There's someone in the staffroom. She looks familiar, though I can't see clearly.

I slump onto the nearest chair.

"Hi Polly." I recognize the voice. It's Moira, one of the parents.

From somewhere a long way off I can hear myself talking. I can't understand the words, they sound like a slowed down tape…

My head's too heavy. I'm falling…

*

I open my eyes. I feel heavy, drugged. I'm lying on my back in a bed. My eyes follow the needle in my right wrist along a thin tube up to a bag from which a colourless liquid drips regularly, like the ticking of a clock. There are wires attached to my chest. I'm linked to a heart monitor.

I'm confused. What happened? What am I doing here? Dennis is sitting beside me staring straight ahead with a cold, angry expression. He doesn't speak as I stir. *Now* I remember…

A short while later Dennis stands. "I have to

get back to the children. I'll come tomorrow." I ask him not to tell the children what I've done. He nods his agreement.

I watch his departing back. I know we won't talk about the overdose. I start to cry from the guilt, the shame, the loss. I didn't want it to be like this for him, for the children, for me...

The one consolation is that Rachel and the boys won't know I've taken an overdose because this is a coronary ward. We're going to hide the truth from them. Tell them Mummy is suffering from exhaustion. Reassure them she'll be better soon.

Chapter Six

Jan's been my counsellor for a year. She's brilliant! One evening a week I settle Joel for sleep then drive the hour it takes to get to her house. She lives in a magnificent Edwardian vicarage in the Lincolnshire Wolds.

My feelings for Jan spiralled out of control long before I realised what was happening. Ironically, I started coming to see her because of the problem with my mother attachment to Sister. After the overdose I was allowed to finish the remaining three months of my teaching contract but then I had to leave the children I loved and the Headteacher who meant so much to me. Now I've replaced one mother figure with another except that this time it's someone who shows me unlimited kindness, compassion and understanding.

Jan smiles when I arrive. She always looks pleased to see me. We go into her kitchen. She makes tea and we take it on a tray to sit in her large, cosy lounge beside a welcoming open fire.

As Jan piles on more coals I watch the flames leaping up the chimney. I feel contented here, bathed in warmth, comforted, loved, like when Mummy lit the fire on late winter afternoons before I started school. We shared many precious moments of closeness then. I knew Mummy cared for me. I was a good girl and she loved me…

Tonight, with Jan, I feel safe, protected again like I used to with Mummy.

"What did you think of Sara?" Jan asks

suddenly. I think back to last week when she took me in her car to a psychologist, the one who supervises her counselling sessions. Jan had told her about my difficulties. Sara thought it would be a good idea if we met. I was extremely anxious when Jan hinted that Sara might be able to help me more than she could but finally accepted her reassurances that she wasn't giving up on me, just exploring different options.

"Sara's nice enough but she's rather cold and distant – not a bit like you."

Jan frowns, looks down at her hands sadly.

Minutes pass without her speaking.

I'm puzzled. We've never experienced an uncomfortable gap in our conversation.

"I'm afraid I've got some bad news for you, Polly," she says quietly.

My stomach lurches. My heart pounds heavily. I know what Jan is going to tell me before she opens her mouth again.

"Sara thinks your problems are too much for me to handle. She says I've become over-involved."

But I can't stop seeing Jan – she's my lifeline. Without her support I can't carry on. We've shared so much, Jan and I – my painful past, my difficulties relating to people, her family problems...

"Jan, I must keep seeing you. You're the one person who helps me to make sense of things."

I wait for a change of expression, a sign that she recognises the need to continue meeting each week. With a sickening, sinking thud I see from her face she's reached a firm decision that I won't be able to alter.

"Polly, I'm sorry. I have to listen to Sara. She's told me that she's willing to see you herself though, so it's not as if you're being left to your own devices."

"I don't want to see Sara," I tell her softly. I sound about six years old. "And that would mean about three hours' driving, there and back. She lives too far away."

But Jan has reached her decision. And the next ten minutes of tearful begging do nothing to shift it.

As usual she hugs me close, wishes me well.

I stand outside her closed door feeling shut out, tempted to knock again but knowing it would make no difference.

My teeth chattering with cold, with shock, I get into my car, place my head on the steering wheel and sob…

Jan satisfied my craving for the motherly concern and interest Mummy can't give me. And it's my stupid fault that the relationship's finished. I've spoilt everything by becoming too needy, too demanding, too emotional to the point where Jan can't take any more…

Now I must be punished. The Little Child in me is terrified, lost, abandoned…

*

It's one of the best days of an English summer.

Sitting beside Joel on a bench on the sea front I'm watching children excitedly floating their boats or paddling in the pool. A light breeze cools the heat of the midday sun. I coped with the loss of Jan initially by throwing myself into supply teaching and now I have a permanent post at a local school. I still get overanxious and, at times, very depressed but I try to hide my problems from everyone, even myself.

My pager bleeps. My heart sinks. Nathan must need an injection. I head for a phone box, ring Dennis.

I know instantly from his cautious tone that he's about to break bad news. An iciness replaces the warmth draining from within me. There's a loud throbbing in my ears. It's difficult to hear him. His words don't make sense. I replay them in my head.

"Rita rang. I'm afraid your mother died an hour ago."

I can't breathe, let alone speak. There's no sun, no seaside, no movement, no sound except Dennis repeating his statement adding, "I'm so sorry, darling."

I'm frozen in time. No emotion. Perhaps it's *me* that's dead.

Dennis is still speaking. I don't understand what he's saying. When he's finished I put down the receiver.

Life has stopped. Her world, my world, both finished, my mind numb, my body paralysed. It's like I've left, gone somewhere else – hearing, seeing, feeling nothing.

I become aware of an insistent tugging at my tee shirt.

"Mummy, can I have an ice-cream?"

Joel doesn't know. I must tell him. "Grandma's died." My voice doesn't belong to me. "She was ill for a long time. Now she's gone to Heaven."

"Yes. Can we go now, Mummy?" I understand his response, his impatience to move on. He hardly knew his grandma. In the past seven years she didn't come to our house. He rarely saw her. I can see why his life isn't devastated by her death as mine is.

I remember the urgent phone-call from Teresa a week ago. "If you want to see Mummy before she goes, you must come soon."

I didn't visit Mummy at Rita's home. It wasn't necessary. Mummy and I had communicated our goodbyes privately, painfully, in the silence of her hospital ward.

I take Joel by the hand. We walk towards the beach.

Anyway, it's not true, I console myself. Deep down inside I don't believe Mummy has gone anywhere. Nobody, nothing, not even death, can defy Mummy.

*

It's several months since I spoke to my Aunt Margaret. And she's important to me now that Aunt Maud , who put me in touch with my real mother, is dead.

I've never met any of Mum's three younger sisters, who live in Ireland but Aunt Maud and I wrote often to each other and spoke regularly on the phone. She listened. She always asked after Dennis and the children and I felt her genuine concern for me.

My Aunt Joan scorned my efforts to maintain contact with her, wouldn't even mention my name in her letters to Mum. I thought it was all to do with me until Mum told me it might be because Joan had disliked her for years. Mum felt that Joan, being the youngest, blamed her for leaving the family home at sixteen, abandoning her as a baby.

Aunt Margaret doesn't ring me. That hurts. Whenever I speak to her it's like talking to a stranger who's only mildly interested in me. But I need her. She's the one blood relative left who has anything to do with me. Even my half-brother shies away from contact with me. Perhaps he feels guilty because he ensured I never inherited the money Mum left me in her will. But I can understand that he might well feel jealous of a thirty-seven–year old big sister who appeared from nowhere, who suddenly disrupted his life. And furthermore, I didn't look for my birth mother for financial gain. I argued in vain against her insistence that I should inherit a part of her fortune after her death.

I dial my aunt's number. Her voice has a coldness to it that makes me shiver. Or am I imagining it?

"How are you?" I ask, knowing she recently had an operation.

"I'm OK," she replies expressionlessly.

Silence.

I'm breaking out in a sweat. She used to

enquire about the children. I don't understand. The tension is unbearable.

"Is there something wrong?" I ask anxiously.

"As a matter of fact there is." She sounds like someone about to make a complaint. "I get Bella delivered every week. I read your article."

My stomach lurches. Suddenly I feel very sick.

"Oh… I see…" is the most I can manage. I'm vividly recalling the article I had published in that women's magazine, revealing the truth about meeting Mum for the first time; the telling phrases like, "Oh God, is that my mother?" and "The house was in a horrendous mess." Those are surely the ones that have offended my aunt. Undoubtedly she's overlooked my expressions of pain at seeing Mum's self-neglect, the reality that I grew to love her, was with her when she died.

"Why didn't you use a false name like one of the other women who wrote about finding her mother?" my aunt asks accusingly. I can't think of an excuse.

Frantically I search for some way to defend myself.

"I understand it must have been horrible for you but magazine editors change things. I didn't write it quite like it came across," I protest weakly.

"Goodbye." My aunt hasn't accepted my attempt to lessen my guilt. She's disgusted at what I wrote. She's rung off.

And she won't ever speak to me again…

I can't deal with this. I feel dirty, sinful. And I must be a thoroughly bad person that both my adoptive and natural families have ended up rejecting me.

Sobbing quietly, I try to cling to the knowledge that Dennis and my children love me unconditionally. But it doesn't reach the Little Girl inside.

She knows she's not good enough for anyone.

*

It's Boxing Day. I've slipped away to my tiny attic study.

I don't want to infect my family with my desperation, dampen their high spirits. I've no right to spoil their fun. I'd feel guilty if I told them what's going on in my head, then watch worried expressions replace their smiles, their laughter, their chatter.

It's impossible to think my own thoughts, to be myself at this moment. Mummy's voice is continually in my mind, fighting to be heard, coaxing, persuasive, demanding, forceful; but always persistent, determined to be listened to. I'm convinced she won't give up until I respond.

Her burial didn't allow her or me any respite or peaceful release. Her power over life didn't end when her body died. Her heart ceased beating but the energy of her mind, the strength of her will, continue to pump through me. She is attempting to achieve what she wants for herself.

And in her final years, she was insistent that she wanted her name on the gravestone before her sister's. The conflict between the two continued to the bitter end. I can't believe they lie peacefully together. Auntie Elise died shortly before Mummy. Three years later, her name is engraved in gold lettering under Daddy's. But there's an empty space between them: Mummy's name is missing.

Mummy refuses to accept her unmarked grave.

Last week I rang the parish priest at the church where she played the organ for over sixty years.

"Nothing to do with us – it's between you and your sisters," he told me.

I tried the funeral director.

"I simply acted on your sister's instructions," he said.

"But you haven't even spelt Auntie Elise's name correctly," I protested.

"It was organised by phone. If you want things changed, you'll have to contact your sister. She was responsible for the funeral arrangements."

I've not rung either of my sisters since their decision to exclude me totally from the family inheritance despite Mummy maintaining in her final years that she wanted to put me back in her will. She'd said it could be difficult as a solicitor friend of Rita's was handling the whole affair. The final blow came when Rita didn't invite me to a family church service the night before Mummy's funeral. I still feel terribly rejected.

But I can't get rid of Mummy's voice:

"It's Christmas. Phone them. You mustn't leave it another day."

I dial Teresa's number. She sounds wary after years of no contact. I come quickly to the point.

"Teresa, why isn't Mummy's name on the tombstone?"

She hesitates. "I honestly don't know why, Polly. Rita handled the whole thing." Her voice is barely audible.

We exchange a few awkward pleasantries and I ring off.

I phone Rita. She sounds pleased I've made the first move to break the silence between us, asks about Dennis and the children. Ill at ease, I answer her questions speedily before giving way to exasperation.

"Rita, why, when Mummy left enough money to cover the funeral costs, have you failed to get her name engraved? I know she damaged the three of us in one way or another, but she doesn't deserve this. No one does."

A pause; has she rung off? My heart is thudding loudly. If she's still there, I'm sure she's going to shout at me.

Then a flippant-sounding, "I haven't got round to it yet. It's actually not high on my list of priorities."

My rage spills over. I'm in full flow now.

"How can you say that? It's been three years. You can't leave it like *this!* If you and Teresa have spent the money Mummy left, I'm willing to give one third of the cost to get it done."

Another silence. Finally, a sigh.

"If it means that much to you, I'll get it done in the summer holidays. Goodbye." Her response is quiet, resigned.

That's seven months' time. And there's no guarantee she'll do it *then…*

I mentally address Mummy. "I've done what I

can for you. Please leave me alone. I can do no
more."

Chapter Seven

I have been seeing another counsellor. As usual it's on the NHS. Even if we could afford for me to consult someone privately, I would not suggest that we spend our hard-earned money trying to get help for my mental health problems. More particularly I am beginning to conclude that either help is simply not available to treat people like me or that I am unconsciously putting up blocks to any therapy.

John is such a kind person. He is also a lecturer on mental health issues. This is our sixth and last session. He told me well in advance about the timescale of treatment.

"Why don't you write poetry?" he suggests.

"I've tried but whatever I write is always pretentious. I can't express what I need to say."

Secretly I think he's only suggesting that because all the talking therapy hasn't worked. And today he's going.

He shakes my hand. "I hope things work out for you. I shall now be writing to your GP to ask for you to be referred to someone else. I don't know how long that will be. Take care."

I liked John. He listened to me as I rambled on about my childhood, passed the tissues when I cried as I spoke of my feelings of loss, helplessness, inadequacy…

I walk slowly back home, tell Dennis this therapy's finished.

"Another therapist bites the dust," he says matter-of-factly.

*

Not surprisingly, the waiting list for treatment means that I am once more left to my own resources. I am determined to sort myself out once and for all.

A friend of mine practises hypnotherapy. She decides to try it with me and I throw myself into total co-operation but excessive anxiety makes relaxation difficult. As usual, each time I try a new approach I am convinced that I have found the answer. Just do whatever I'm told and my life will be happy, I will accept and possibly even like myself. Everyone will notice the change in me and this time it will be for real. I won't just be putting on an act of being confident, friendly and outgoing.

That will be the new, changed me.

After several attempts she tells me there's not much point in continuing. "I know you're only pretending each time to be hypnotised, to please me," she announces.

And she's right.

*

I decide to try a different tack. There seem to be hundreds of self-help books being written these days. Books on how to overcome your fears, your depression, your anger, how to meditate, how to stop feeling guilty, how to gain confidence, how to make friends, how to be positive, how to make money, how to...

I not only buy them, I read them and get

animated with the mounting certainty of success as I near the end. I close each book with the conviction that from this moment on I will never again indulge a negative emotion. I then place the life-changing text on my bookshelf, take a long, deep breath and prepare for the wonderful experiences ahead...

*

It's teatime, four hours since I finished reading the last manual that was supposed to help me to turn my life around. Nathan needs an injection for a bleed into his ankle, the washing machine is leaking, Benjamin and Joel are having an argument and Dennis hasn't returned in time for our meal.

The tranquility, the surge of positive intentions, the feeling of goodwill to others as well as myself, so strongly felt just a short while ago, are lost as I rush around trying to calm the chaos around me. I feel fraught, enraged, frenetic and completely inadequate.

*

I've tried a number of different anti-depressants but drastic side effects, which leave me feeling physically ill, always deter me from continuing. I've taken a variety of herbal remedies for anxiety and depression. They fail to have the desired effect. And with no other help on offer from the medical profession at present, I'm at my wits end. I can't deal with the way I seem to lurch from one crisis to the next, with the sad happenings in friends' lives that leave me feeling unhappy for them and powerless to help, with the pent-up feelings that Dennis refuses to share with me about our marriage and his own problems. I must get some other help, try to make things better for all our sakes.

I phone a Life Coach, hearing the desperate edge to my voice as I bargain with him for a reduced fee to attend his workshops and meditation classes.

*

I have attended regularly. I'm punctual for every lesson of the course on how to radically change my thinking, to wholeheartedly change my life.

Everything I'm being taught makes good sense, there is nothing to dispute. The method is speedy, foolproof and predictable if you take the time to listen and internalise the auditory and visual messages. You can change your thinking and therefore your life. By merely altering my body language, choosing to fill my mind with uplifting thoughts and creating positive goals for myself I can totally reframe my approach to myself, to my relationships, to my life. I can feel good emotionally and spiritually. It's simply a choice I need to make. It's that easy…

So why am I hidden away in my attic study trying to hide my distress from my family? I feel so ignorant, pathetic, guilty and angry with myself. I'm am as negative inside as before, despite all the wonderful ideas I'm passing onto my children every night when we're gathered round the table for the family meal.

Only one thing has changed. I no longer blame anyone else for my distress. I am an adult, I am no longer a child, an innocent victim of the abuse I suffered. I now take full responsibility for who I am, what I think and do. I also think that I am somehow responsible for anything that has happened to me, which means in no uncertain terms that I am a thoroughly bad person who deserves all the horrible things that have happened in my life.

Chapter Eight

This afternoon the school secretary phoned me at home. I'd returned to school after several months' absence recovering from an operation.

Trying to cope without support with the special needs class of socially-deprived and severely emotionally-disturbed six-year-olds proved too much for me. Within days I was off with back pain, so excruciating I was unable to get out of bed. I've never had a back problem in my life. When the doctor visited she examined me before saying, "I think your body is trying to tell you something." I didn't understand what she meant.

I am due to return later this week and now I am informed that the Head has asked for me to see. I strongly suspect that she wishes to begin disciplinary action against me for my time off work. I know from past experience that I have achieved unpopularity by my outspoken views on the current pressures on teachers, by sympathising with a newly qualified, stressed- out teacher who, heavily criticised by the Head and staff, was driven to resign.

At some level I know I am a competent teacher, but I can't cope with twenty-four mentally and behaviourally challenging children in a classroom on my own. I'm not trained to deal with the complexities involved in this sort of specialized teaching. Yesterday I anonymously phoned a counselor in the Education Department who told me categorically that prolonged absence due to stress would result in suspension and eventual dismissal.

I also phoned my union representative who agreed that, given the circumstances, my best option is to take early retirement on health grounds. My G.P. has already mentioned that it's possible she can help me to leave in this way, by virtue of years of frequent, recurrent depression. But, nevertheless, to me it spells failure.

This feels like a repetition of my experience in Canada. I'm no good at anything, no use to anyone. I can't stay in this mess I've created. There must be a way out. I'm on the verge of losing my mind. I've got to do something, anything…

I grab cleaning materials from the cupboard, frenetically clean every light switch in the house in a desperate effort to rid myself of the mental images of impending disaster. Dennis' pleas for me to slow down fall on deaf ears. I know this isn't helping me but I no longer feel in control. I feel compelled to do something drastic. I ring the psychiatric ward of our local hospital where after much pleading, I speak to a psychiatrist who agrees to see me later in the day.

But first I have another appointment to keep.

The psychologist I have been seeing on a weekly basis is attempting to use Cognitive Behaviour Therapy – a treatment designed to replace my negative thinking with a more constructive approach through awareness and restructuring of my thought processes. However, the hour is invariably taken up with my latest confrontation with the Headmistress or my frequent crises of confidence whenever an inspector or another teacher observes my lessons. Even excellent Ofsted reports on my teaching have done little to dispel the steady loss of confidence in my teaching ability over the last eight years. If the Head of the school does not praise my efforts then to me they are futile, worthless.

After listening to my distress Marcus leans forward in his chair, urges me gently but firmly to go to the hospital immediately. He knows I have reached my limit, is aware that I can no longer tolerate the avalanche of negative emotions. I need more help than he is able to give me and I need it now before it is too late…

*

I've been incarcerated for three months in a side room of this acute ward.

I'm a voluntary patient. I could leave this psychiatric unit at any time. But I no longer know how to take responsibility for myself. The pressures of teaching were too great. The tenuous coping with the job, with my life, snapped at that particular point.

I hate myself. I'm pathetic. I've failed completely, utterly. I'm no use to myself or anyone else.

The doctor prescribed sedatives, sleeping medication and an anti-depressant called Venlafaxine. "It helps a lot of people," he said.

But it didn't suit me. Increasingly confused, angry and depressed I resorted to impulsive episodes of self-harm and overdosing. I've become skilful at escaping past locked doors into town to find respite in over-the-counter pills and alcohol.

I was given a different mind-altering drug.

"Seroxat is extremely effective in relieving depression," the doctor reassured me.

But the situation has worsened. The pit I'm in is darker, deeper. I search constantly for some form of relief. This morning I went into a utility room, smashed a glass vase and used the shards to slash at my hands until blood flowed freely, covering the floor. It didn't hurt one bit.

"My God!" exclaimed a nurse who spotted me silently immersed in releasing some of the pent-up rage that could find no other outlet. She rushed in with several towels, removed the glass from my grasp, wrapped the towels round my hands. I watched the bright liquid soaking into the white fabric. At her request I accompanied her to the nurses' office, where I smeared blood angrily onto the walls.

"Oh, look! There's blood everywhere! What a colourful design!" I announced sarcastically to my astonished audience. I was given another tranquilliser. But they've long ceased to have any effect.

It's dinnertime. As usual I can't make myself eat the bland-looking food. The smell is bad enough. Whilst nursing-staff are occupied serving meals, I slip out of the ward, seizing the opportunity as a porter opens the door to come in. I'll need to be quick though, before anyone notices my disappearance.

I run to the nearest car park. I don't know why

I'm doing this…

A middle-aged woman is about to get into her car.

I glance over my shoulder. No one's following me but I know there's not much time.

"Are you going near Tesco's?" I ask breathlessly, keeping my bandaged hands well hidden from sight. She turns, looks surprised.

I don't wait for a reply. "I've been visiting my mother in hospital but I'm running late. I promised I'd meet a friend half an hour ago."

"I'm not going that way," she says bluntly.

"Well, could you give me a lift to the main road? That would save me time," I say urgently, hoping she won't see my panic.

"I'm not sure about this." She sounds uncomfortable. "I'm already late for my round to see patients. I don't like giving lifts."

"I'd be really grateful. I don't want to disappoint my friend," I persist.

She hesitates before relenting. "All right – get in then." I hear the note of annoyance but I don't care that she's not happy.

I want to urge her to hurry but somewhere at the back of my head I know that would make her suspicious. And I'm not going to be shamed by being marched back to the ward.

We don't talk. She stops the car. I thank her. She drives off.

Another car pulls in to the kerb. Someone is dropping his girlfriend off.

"Could you possibly give me a lift into town?" I ask the driver. I keep my hands behind my back.

"No problem." He's obligingly friendly.

Seated beside him I work out exactly what I'm going to do…

He drops me off in the centre of town. My plan absorbs every ounce of concentration. It's exciting to know exactly what will happen next. And so far it's working well. I'm in control.

I go into the chemist's, buy a couple of packets of travel pills, pocket them and head single-mindedly for my next port of call – the wine merchant's. I select the first bottle of vodka I come to, pay for it and book a taxi from a public phone box, to meet me outside the shopping complex in ten minutes time. That's how long I think I'll need to go into the public toilet and carry out my secret plan…

Fortunately there's no one else here. I wash the tablets down with the strong-tasting alcohol, not allowing the bitter taste to linger in my mouth.

I shudder. Already I can feel the effect. I'm starting to drift. My body is relaxing. I'm losing focus…

I must hurry. It's like walking through treacle. But I can't face the disgrace of collapsing in broad daylight in front of passing shoppers.

I feel sick. My feet don't seem to want to go in the direction of the taxi. The black vehicle is waiting.

From somewhere far off, a voice says, "Where to?"

I fall onto the back seat. "The County Hospital." My tongue feels too large, the words are slurring.

I close the door. There's a whirring in my ears.

I feel numb. Sight, sounds are receding further, further…

No one, nothing, matters…

*

It's Christmas Day. The normally overcrowded ward is practically empty. A decorated tree is the one sign that this day is different from any other. There are only a few patients unable to go home for the festive season. I wish I had the courage to leave, to get out and never come back. I'm not getting better. A psychiatrist checks on my current state once a week. There is no therapy, no treatment, simply medication and a locked door. I can see no end to this half-life. If it weren't for the pastel pictures I have started doing, I'm sure I would lose all sense of reality. I mainly do them to fill the endless empty hours and because others like the results, encourage me to do more. Dennis brings in photos of our summer holiday in Venice and I try to recreate the warmth of the scenes, the atmosphere, hoping that some of it will rub off on me. But deep inside I feel dead.

Dennis and the children are spending the afternoon with me. It is cramped in this small room I've been allotted for their visit. For the first time ever we are unsure of what to say to each other. I feel so guilty about what my illness is doing to my family, especially the children. And today is the first time Joel has set foot inside the unit. Usually I meet him outside and he, Dennis and I go out for a meal. I feel I have abandoned my fourteen-year-old at a vulnerable age, at a time when he still needs me. I was there for him all through his life until now. None of the children know quite what to say seeing me like this. It's a tremendous shock for them. They are used to a strong, confident, coping mum. The conversation is strained, awkward, forced. My talk, my laughter sounds false, hollow and convinces no one.

On the way out Nathan, who's twenty, takes me to one side. He looks me straight in the eyes.

"Mum you have no idea what you look like. You are shuffling about in your slippers with your shoulders bent and your head down. You look like some old woman. Get a grip of yourself. Hold yourself up, walk straight, talk to the other patients. You can do it if you make up your mind."

He kisses me warmly. I understand his anger.

I watch them go. I've let my family down. They did nothing to deserve to see their mum in this bleak prison for lost souls. Returning to my room I throw myself on the bed and sob.

*

"You've got visitors," the nurse says. "In the office."

Nathan's haematologist and Dennis are standing near the door. They both look very serious. In spite of my drugged stupor I sense immediately that something is dreadfully wrong.

"What's happened? Where's Nathan?"

Dennis puts a hand on my shoulder. "Just listen

to what the doctor has to say."

The doctor comes straight to the point. "One of the donors to a recent batch of the Factor VIII given to Nathan for his injections died from CJD. That means there is a theoretical chance that Nathan could have been infected." His words are a harsh contrast to the soft, kind tone of his voice.

"Oh no!" I cup my hand over my mouth, feel my legs giving way. Dennis guides me to a chair. I sit sobbing, convinced that my handsome son who managed to escape HIV infection is now going to die of CJD.

The doctor is speaking again. I force myself to listen.

"There is as yet no proven risk of transmission of the disease through blood but we can't rule it out. I've already phoned Nathan to tell him."

Nathan is in Spain for a year with his girlfriend. I can't even be there to comfort him. I'm hurting too much. This can't be happening. It can't be real. Through the noise of my crying, I can hear the doctor's voice.

"Nathan asked me what the news meant. I told him that in twenty or thirty years there's a remote possibility that he could contract the disease."

I can't bear this. It must have been horrible for Nathan. He must be in a terrible state.

"What did he say? How is he?"

"He took it extremely well. He simply thanked me for telling him and said, 'Now I'll get on with the rest of my life.' "

I'm trying to take in what I've heard. I'm so relieved Nathan didn't panic. And if he's taken the

news so calmly what right do I have to fall apart
over it?

*

This brief encounter with the outside world has
jerked me back into some form of rational
thought...

And I have one small consolation in the midst
of this nightmarish existence: I've been granted
early retirement from teaching. I'll never have to
return to the profession I once loved but which
hastened my downfall in recent years.

Yet only the standard written acknowledgement
from the Education Department marks the end of
my teaching career. There is no customary leaving
present from the staff of the school where I taught
for the last eight years, no letter of thanks from the
Head, not even a get well card...

I feel completely undeserving, totally rejected.

*

This halfway house has been my home for
nearly two months.

On my arrival I was informed of its purpose: to
provide a transition for me, and others like me, from
the acute psychiatric ward to living a normal life in
society.

There's no therapy here. We're left completely
to our own devices. Each resident is given a weekly
sum of money for food. I must shop and cook for

myself.

I'm not hungry. No one checks whether I eat or not. With each passing hour my feeling of helplessness intensifies. The other residents rarely speak except to pass the time of day. Staff chat mainly amongst themselves, taking scant interest in us.

The lounge in this decrepit old house has a constant haze of cigarette smoke hanging in the air. Most of the staff and residents congregate here to puff away the hours, days, weeks, speaking intermittently, sometimes not at all.

I hate sitting in this smoke-filled room but it's a stark choice: this, or remain alone in my bedroom upstairs, isolated from the world.

My medication has been increased to include a drug that has the effect of giving continuous jolts of electricity through my body. No amount of insisting that I can't live with this sensation makes the slightest difference to medical staff. They think it's my imagination.

Inmates look sorely neglected. There's John, over by the window. In his twenties, he's spent five years here already. Lost in his own world he mumbles incessantly to himself, doesn't appear to be aware of anything, anybody. And poor Olive, who's in her early forties but looks much older, can't sit still. She approaches a member of staff, complains about something. Cross at being ignored she shuffles noisily round the room in her down-at-heel slippers inhaling, almost without pausing, on the cigarette between her nicotine-stained fingers.

She shakes constantly from head to foot. Olive has spent the last ten years in this place.

Martin's just come in. As usual he's wearing that angry expression of his. He says nothing, merely projects some of his repressed rage, glowering fiercely at me until I shrink further into my chair, terrified in case he erupts into uncontrolled verbal or physical abuse. For twelve years he's been pacing this shabby room. His enormous bulk and bushy grey beard seem to emphasise his silent fury at the world.

If I stay here I'll become one of them. There's nothing halfway about this institution – it's a dead end. Difficult patients are left here to rot until death or some other fate befalls them. I'm not going to end up blubbering like John, whining and jittery like Olive, an unexploded time-bomb like Martin. I refuse to be relegated to the shadowy world of these mentally sick souls, to join the sad outcasts, the misfits of our country's mental health system. I'm not well enough to go home but I'm not staying here a second longer. I know how to escape. I'm here on condition that I don't self-harm...

I put on my coat, walk down the hill into town, order a taxi. I buy painkillers, alcohol, go into a toilet to overdose myself into oblivion...

I'm feeling better already. Confidently I get into the waiting taxi, tell the driver my destination and fight the urge to close my eyes, to sleep. I watch pedestrians who appear to be swaying from one side of the pavement to the other...

The car screeches to a halt. I hold out money to the driver but I can't see his face. He puts change in my hand.

I stagger up the slope to the house. I never realised how steep it is. In the entrance Dennis and a friend are staring anxiously at me. I open my mouth to speak but the words don't come.

"Get an ambulance!" somebody shouts in the distance.

My legs won't hold my weight. The hallway is spinning violently.

I don't care what happens next...

*

My punishment for the overdose is a further spell in another acute ward back in the County Hospital. My Primary Nurse, who is supposed to work out a care plan for my stay is the exact opposite of Maria on the other ward. Her lack of interest in me is so evident that I only became aware I was assigned to her when she passed me a note suggesting we find a time to discuss my future but that right now she was too busy.

Dennis is beside me as I approach her this afternoon with my worry about the violent-looking patient who appears to follow me wherever I go and seems to delight at farting close to me. I begin to tell her my concerns but halfway through my sentence, with no warning, she transfers her attention to another nurse who has just walked in to talk to her.

I turn to Dennis. "Is it my imagination or has she just switched me off?"

"You're not imagining anything. That's

precisely what she did." There is a look of amazement on his face. Rudeness is one trait in others that he finds inexcusable.

"Right, I'm not putting up with this," I say angrily. "I'm leaving, I'm going now." She shows no sign that she's heard me.

Leaving Dennis to explain I go to pack my bags.

The doctor is called. He consents. I'm free to leave if I think I can handle my life.

The air feels cool, fresh on my hot face as we walk out into the spring evening.

*

There are some events that took place when I was in the acute ward that, probably because of the large cocktail of prescribed drugs, I cannot remember. Most of that eight-month period is a fog through which I can see only the odd scene with clarity.

Dennis has told me about other episodes like when I hid behind a food trolley in the dining room terrified to come out in case my father spanked me. There was the heated argument that I insisted was taking place across my bed between my adoptive mother and my birth mother. "They won't leave me alone!" I shrieked to Dennis on the phone.

Dennis says that on another occasion I rang him pleading for the phone number of my real mother in the U.S.A. Ignoring his reminder that I was with her when she died, I continued to beg for her number saying that she was there by my side, asking me to ring her.

One day I apparently decided to protect myself by taking the decision not to speak to anyone. It seems I kept my promise for five days.

And a few incidents are like clips remembered from a film seen years ago:

One night I hid for hours under my bed shaking, petrified that my father would find me, drag me out and beat me.

Another time I came to on a bed, wanting to go to the toilet. It was, I found out later, after one of the six overdoses I took whilst hospitalised. I recall heading for the toilet, missing the door and hearing a very loud bang like a gunshot as I made contact with the wall. Putting my hand to my face I was surprised that considering the amount of blood, I felt no pain. My whole body was numb. Perhaps the accident jolted me into some state of awareness as the horrified exclamations of nurses who came running towards me, presumably because they'd heard the noise, are imprinted on my brain. I should like to think that the black eyes and bruised, swollen forehead served as a reminder to staff that I should not have been left alone.

Then there was the night in the secure observation room that I banged for hours as hard as I could on the Perspex-covered windows, not relenting until after several injections I finally collapsed onto the mattress on the floor.

Chapter Nine

I should be feeling great. It's five months since I was in hospital. I'm on holiday on a campsite in Italy with blues skies, hot sunny weather, wonderful scenery and glorious beaches. I'm also on the maximum dose of the anti-depressant, Seroxat. So I can't understand why I'm so miserable. And the relaxed, smiling faces of other holidaymakers emphasise the darkness of my depression. Surrounded by people I feel cut off, desolate, deeply unhappy. These tablets are obviously not working.

I consult the campsite doctor, who agrees that the tablets are not helping and tells me how to slowly decrease the medication day by day.

*

We are at the end of the long coach journey home. Yesterday I took my final tablet. I am walking as though in a dream, not from tiredness alone but from the certainty that this dark hole I've fallen into is where I shall stay unless I can somehow release myself.

I leave my suitcase in the porch, go to my room and fill a beaker with water in the en suite. I take a bottle of tablets out of the cabinet and swallow handfuls of them. I'm on automatic pilot with no thought about what I'm doing.

In an instant I feel very frightened. I look at the bottle. It's almost empty . I've no idea how many pills I've taken. I can feel the panic rising. What am I doing? I didn't mean it to end like this. My hand is shaking violently as I dial Marcus's number.

I recognize the gentle tone of his voice. "Marcus," I say through my tears, "I've taken an overdose. Please help me."

In the distance I can hear him saying. "Pass me onto your husband."

Dennis has just walked into the room. I hand him the receiver. The world goes black...

*

While the rest of the world was reeling from events unfolding in America on September 11th, 2001, I was once again recovering in the acute ward, oblivious to the events that had shattered the lives of so many people...

It was a week before I surfaced enough to take a long look at myself and those around me – sad, bewildered creatures closed off in our drugged, tormented minds. Staying here, surrounded by the tortured faces of others, steeped in my own misery and wallowing in shame could hardly be a recipe for recovery. If I didn't get out fast this time I realised that I might never have the courage to pick up the pieces of my life again.

I rang Dennis. "Can you please collect me. I'm coming home."

*

I pull my coat my coat closely round me, perch nervously on the edge of my seat.

It's nine months since I walked out of the acute ward, determined to move forward, leave the past behind, make a fresh start. I must never allow myself to get that bad again. Nathan's words to me strengthened that resolve. We were sitting together in the conservatory shortly after my discharge from hospital when he said, "Mum, I don't think you have any idea how it feels to have a mother who has tried to take her own life."

But depression washes over me in waves, the temptation to destroy myself is getting harder to resist, a sense of hopelessness is threatening to spoil my attempts to lead some kind of normal life. An inner desperation and loneliness conflict with the happy front I put on for the benefit of those around me. Who, after all, wants to spend too much time in the company of someone who complains about the way they feel, whose long face brings down the tone of a social occasion, who is self-centred, self-absorbed?

I've had a few appointments with this consultant psychiatrist. And he has prescribed one anti-depressant after another in the hope of finding something that works for me. I've had enough of being fobbed off, I intend to make my feelings clear.

"So how are you? " he asks without moving his chair away from his desk.

"I'm no better, Doctor. I have short periods when things are OK and I try to ignore the depression when it begins, but it sweeps over me and I seem powerless to deal with it."

"Right, let's see, which anti-depressants

haven't we tried?"

I knew this would happen. He's thinking of giving me yet another lot of tablets with horrible side effects. And so it will continue if I don't change the pattern.

"I'm not taking another anti-depressant, Doctor. They make me feel awful. I can't stand them."

"Well, I'm afraid there's nothing more I can offer you, Mrs Fielding. And now I have another patient to see."

He's clearly annoyed at what he perceives as my non-co-operation. He's sending me away with no hint of recovery. How dare he think he can get rid of me on this note of dismissal!

I feel a mixture of anger, fear and excitement rising within me.

"I'm not leaving here until you do something different to help me, Doctor."

"Mrs Fielding, I have already given you fifteen minutes of my time and I have a lot of other patients to see." I can hear the irritation in his voice. But I'm not about to give up now.

"I'm not moving from this room until you suggest something more helpful." I'm trembling and stunned by my audacity in challenging someone in his position. But I'm full of despair, I need to find a way out before I lose control and do something destructive to myself. "I mean what I say, I'm going to sit right here until you offer me something more constructive." I can hear the decisiveness in my voice, I just wish I felt as confident as I sound.

The doctor is silent. He fiddles with his tie. He looks out of the window. Now he's arranging the papers on his desk. Perhaps he's hoping that by ignoring me I'll decide to leave. But I can't give up now. Shaking all over, I watch his changes of expression. He's beginning to look extremely uncomfortable, keeps shifting position in his chair.

Time seems to stand still. My heart is pounding. The silence between us is tense, threatening, terrifying.

His loud voice makes me jump. "I'm asking you one last time to leave my office, Mrs Fielding."

He sounds really angry.

"No," I say, feeling as I used to when, having defied Daddy, I was at the point where I knew he would put me across his knee and beat me senseless.

The doctor picks up the phone, asks someone to come immediately.

A tall man enters the room.

"Do you have a problem, Doctor?"

"This patient is refusing to leave my office. I've asked her several times."

"I'm the manager of this department, the doctor has told you the session is finished so I'm asking you to leave this building now. You are keeping other patients waiting."

"Why should I leave when the doctor is suggesting nothing except tablets that don't work? I am desperate for help." But I feel intimidated.

"Have you made your diagnosis, Doctor?" he asks.

"Yes, There's nothing I can do. There isn't

even any room in the wards to admit her."

I'm outnumbered. But I make one last plea, thinly disguised by my defiant tone.

"So, you won't help me? What are you going to do? Are you going to get the police to throw me out?" I address my question to the manager.

"If it comes to it, yes."

I've never been in trouble with the law before and I don't want to make things even worse by forcing them to take this course of action,

"Well, you obviously have no intention of doing anything for me so my staying here a moment longer is pointless."

I stand, attempt to look dignified, turn and walk towards the door holding on to the remote hope that the doctor will try to make it easier for me. But I know that this particular battle to get help for myself has ended with me looking rather foolish.

*

Perhaps the doctor had second thoughts when I left him that day. Whatever the reason, he referred me for a completely different type of therapy, one that was popular after the second world war to treat shell-shocked soldiers. Therapeutic Communities were set up to enable patients to gain insight into their problems through living and working together, talking about their difficulties and, with mutual feedback, to replace destructive coping mechanisms with positive ones.

Chapter Ten

I feel old, tired. I've had enough of anger, despair, self-pity, neediness and self-hatred. In this Therapeutic Community, where I live from Monday to Friday, we are encouraged to feel and express emotions.

I have had too much backlash from expressing mine. It is often in the form of attack, like the verbal fury that was unleashed when I tried to rid myself of my pent-up anger by deliberately walking into brambles until my legs were scratched and bleeding. I tried to hide what I'd done but I'd been noticed in the garden by another resident. I was so ashamed and unhappy.

I am seen as unco-operative, defensive. So now I play the game, listening to others, rarely speaking in the twice-daily hour-long Whole Community meetings and twice–weekly Small Group meetings when six of us and a couple of staff members discuss more in-depth issues. On occasion I give feedback in an attempt to help others gain an understanding of why they feel as they do. I have identified with much of the abuse they've suffered. But I'm twenty years older than anyone else here. They have never been parents, had children, so how can they possibly understand what that feels like?

Why is there no consistent feedback from staff? Perhaps people can learn to understand what triggers their present feelings and behaviour; but how do they move on?

'Sit with the feelings' seems to be the motto. Yet no coping mechanisms are taught to manage those feelings, to attempt to live and behave differently. Past therapies have made me realise *why* I react to people and situations in an inappropriate manner. But that does not help me to cope, to change…

*

MAGGIE'S TAKEN OVERDOSE SLEEPING TABLETS TRANQUILLISERS PAINKILLERS WAITING FOR HER TO CALL AMBULANCE DON'T KNOW ADDRESS

This text has just come through on my mobile from a fellow resident. A tidal wave of powerful emotion surges through me. I'm angry. Every weekend our telephone support network requires residents of our Therapeutic Community to be on call twenty-four hours a day. During the week we live and work together and staff are on hand for such emergencies as this. But Saturdays and Sundays they're only available for a few hours a day. How unfair a delegation of responsibility is this? We're not trained in crisis management. We're caught up in our own problems yet we can't ignore a desperate plea from any member of the Community. The onus is on us to respond appropriately. And if someone succeeds in taking their own life, where does that leave the rest of us?

For the past half-hour I've been trying to decide whether I should have pressurised Maggie so hard last week to face up to her vulnerability. I've even rehearsed the tack I'll take this week to force her to speak, to deal with her own issues instead of using massive avoidance tactics.

I grudgingly admire Maggie. She reminds me of my sister Rita when we were young. She's popular, attractive, young, articulate, intelligent, witty and strong-minded – everything *I* would like to be. She's very selective about her friends. She rarely speaks to me outside meetings.

After seven months in the Community, Maggie commands a high level of respect for her leadership and consistently helpful feedback in meetings. Her overdose feels like blanket permission for the rest of us to self-harm when the fancy takes us.

"Pile on the pressure," she urged me recently.

"We're really very alike, you and me." So I did. I too am expert at manipulation, deceit and finding endless ways to avoid facing my emotions head on.

I want to escape the burden of guilt, the frustration, fear, trauma, grief… and above all, the jealousy.

A part of me is terribly upset about what she has done and wants to be there for her, to do anything I can to make her feel better. I know she would not want to see me, would resent any attempt I might make to understand, to share her desperation, her unhappiness. I feel useless, inadequate, rejected…

As for the staff…! I want to rage at them for the lack of twenty-four hour cover for just such an emergency. Being left to deal with this alone, not knowing where other members of the Community are, geographically or emotionally, is cruel. We don't have the resources or the knowledge to cope. We can't even call an ambulance on another's behalf.

It's enough dealing with myself. I don't need this...

*

This morning I lost my ring.

It was a special ring. I took ages choosing it whilst on holiday in Greece. It was too tight when I first tried it on. After the jeweller enlarged it, I spent hours agonising that it might fall off when my hands were cold. Eventually I plucked up courage to return and request that it be reduced in size.

I was delighted with my present to myself. It fitted my little finger perfectly. The gold zigzag design is supposed to represent the ups and downs of life. So appropriate! When I was depressed it would remind me that things get better.

It must have slipped off when I dried my hands on the coarse paper towels we have here. But the dustman came shortly before I began my search so my desperate rummage through the bins was futile.

I'm sure I didn't leave it at home. But I rang Dennis anyway and asked him to check the pockets of my clothes.

"I'll buy you another one to make up for it," he offers, kindly.

I find an empty room, build a barricade of chairs and lie down behind them...

Someone has found me, covered me with a

sheet. I pull it over my head. Tears do nothing to relieve the frustration and an overwhelming sense of loss. It's like I've lost a part of me…

The white mark on my finger is a sad reminder of something important that I had and lost. I feel hurt, deprived. An act of kindness to myself wiped out in a few seconds.

"It's only a ring," I say over and over in my head and to anyone who'll listen.

But I'm distraught. I can't eat, can't sleep. Even medication hasn't calmed me.

*

"Nine o'clock meeting open. Written clinical feedback from staff. It's bad news, I'm afraid."

We listen intently. The Chairperson reads solemnly.

"We've been informed by the acute ward that Bill has taken his life…"

My stomach sinks. A wave of fury spreads rapidly through my body. My nightmare has become reality. I prayed so hard this wouldn't happen.

Impulsively I stand, turn towards the door.

Firm voices urge me to stay. They won't accept my desire to run. I storm from the room, engulfed by a terrible rage, pace back and forth in the dining area.

Why didn't someone hear me two months ago, while there was still time to save him? I told them *then* that we allowed him to go home to die.

I remember with fondness the gentle-natured

old fellow, his bewildered eyes bloodshot from years of drinking, peering at the world through thick-lensed glasses, his balding head a stark contrast to the dense mass of grey beard covering his face. He wore the same clothes every day. He'd lost interest in his appearance, in himself. The narrow conservatory would fill with smoke as he puffed on his pipe, reminiscing about the past…

Another resident interrupts my thoughts.

"I've been asked to tell you to return."

Reluctantly I comply. Back in the meeting room my anger erupts. I let rip, hold nothing back.

"I'm fucking furious!" I shout. " Not with residents – with staff! They were asked to deal with the issue of Bill's personal hygiene. Because they ignored it, residents tackled it badly, telling him he smelt. He couldn't handle it…!"

"Your anger is understandable," the psychotherapist remarks calmly. "But what could we have done? It was his decision to leave."

I'm incensed by this denial of staff responsibility. "You could have put things in place for him. You knew his little dog was the only creature in the world he felt cared about him. I used to ring him at weekends, try to persuade him to consider how much his dog depended on him – how he wouldn't survive without his owner. But it wasn't enough. *You* could have done something else. You could have put him in touch with other services that could help him…"

"We let his G.P. know."

"He needed *more!* We let him down. *We let him die!*"

"His life was his responsibility," a resident reminds me sharply.

I've started on my angry roller coaster. It's going to take a lot to shut me up. "I know that! But you have to be extremely strong to stay here. Don't I know about *that!*" I hear the bitterness creeping in as I remember the times I've been targeted for angry feelings of other residents.

"Bill wasn't strong enough – he couldn't take it! Staff weren't prepared to step in."

"You always have to blame someone, don't you? If it isn't residents, it's staff."

I'm undeterred by this resident's attempt to protect the professionals.

"Staff are accountable. This should never have happened," I tell her.

"Fuck off!" she shrieks, striding from the room.

I make a move to leave.

"You need to stay!" a chorus of voices tell me.

"We knew you'd be angry," says a staff member. "Everyone needs to talk about this."

"No amount of talk will bring Bill back!" I say sullenly. I flop back in my chair, defeated.

The next part of the session is taken up with others' expressions of anger, shame, guilt, sadness about their own lives…

I stay silent. It's pointless to say another word.

Gavin is talking about his relationships with past and present girlfriends.

Gazing through the window at trees in the distance, I no longer hear what he's saying. I'm thinking about Bill. Poor, unhappy, friendless Bill, his fight for life lost at the age of sixty-four.

There are fourteen other people sitting here, their eyes fixed on the floor. As for me, I'm far away in a place where no one can reach me.

*

In six days time this therapy finishes. I will have spent a year in this large, old, rundown house, going home only for weekends. Every day I have to watch my back. No one is allowed to launch a physical attack but some of the verbal onslaughts during our daily two hour-long meetings have caused many of us tears of hurt and humiliation. Residents behave like children which, to my shame, includes me. Any so-called offence is punished by a mass, often silently agreed, punishment. If a resident says or does something that annoys the Community, being ignored by everyone is one of the milder consequences. Yet we are supposed to talk freely, uninhibitedly. When one lad, in his twenties, talked about his sexual deviations he was given the cold shoulder by some and subjected to snide, cruel remarks from others. We often act like children – cuddling soft toys for comfort, regarding the staff as parents and having a party with games like 'pass the parcel' the night before a resident leaves.

They're furious because I have decided not to have a party. I've spoilt things for everyone, I've been told. But I can't stand anything like that. I'm happy to accept the customary parting gift – I've already opted for a plant. It will look good in the conservatory of the bungalow we've just bought.

And I have no objection to choosing the menu for my last meal here either. But I am not going to force myself to dress up, play silly games and pretend to be having a good time.

I'm leaving with a lot of anger – about Bill, about a member of staff who has become yet another mother figure in my eyes (something I scarcely dare admit to myself let alone the Community), about the fact that we all have severe problem here yet we are supposed to find solutions by challenging each other. Staff never give guidance on a one-to-one basis and rarely intervene in Group meetings. Yet two nurses have left because they were unhappy here and a further two are off with stress.

This weekend I shall be going to our new home for the first time. I scoured the house last Sunday, collecting every diazepam tablet I could find, hidden in cupboards all over the place. I've got a completely full bottle of high-strength tranquillisers.

I told Dennis I was taking them with me for safekeeping so Joel wouldn't find them. Though, as Dennis rightly stated, "Joel won't take them." If things get too uncomfortable for me I'll just take one every now and then to make myself feel better…

And I am a lot better. I now voice my opinions strongly without worrying whether people will dislike me. I feel more confident in myself and it will be a relief to get out of this place and go on the booked holiday to Spain the day after I leave. My family and friends have all remarked on the positive changes in me.

I breathe a sigh of relief as the morning meeting ends. The room is hot and stuffy, I long to taste freedom again, to walk along a sandy beach in the hot sunshine.

A nurse stops me on my way to make coffee. "There's a phone call for you."

I go into the cramped little room, with graffiti scrawled on the walls, that serves as a telephone booth.

I pick up the receiver. The moment Dennis speaks I can hear he's worried. I know he wasn't feeling well yesterday. "How are you?" I ask.

"Haven't they told you?" he says.

"Told me what?"

"I spoke to a member of staff a short while ago asking them to break the news to you that we had a burglary last night."

I'm stunned. I can't think straight. I say nothing.

"Everything was packed up downstairs ready for the removal firm coming today. Joel and I were asleep when it happened. We didn't hear a thing. They've stolen a lot of our stuff."

I feel sick. "What about my natural mother's rings?"

"I think they've gone. When I came down this morning the first thing I noticed was your jewellery box open on the table. I'd left it on top of the computer. That's gone too."

My mind is whirring like a machine out of control.

"I can't handle this, I'll get one of the staff."

I leave the receiver hanging, go directly to the

staff room, knock and enter without waiting for an answer.

Three faces are staring at me, surprised at my sudden intrusion into their meeting.

"Dennis has just told me we've been burgled. They've taken my mother's rings." The words come out in a breathless rush.

"Sit down," the psychotherapist says.

I do as I'm told but I'm finding it more and more difficult to think clearly. My brain is clogged up. Waves of panic keep sweeping over me. My one hope is that the staff will help me to get through this.

"Please give me something strong to calm me down," I beg. "I can't cope with this. It's too much for me."

"Polly, listen carefully. We will consider giving you something later on but for now I want you to go to the Small Group meeting, which is starting in five minutes. You can talk there about what has happened."

"You don't understand." I can hear the whine. I can't control the rising pitch of my voice. I can feel every bit of self-control slipping away rapidly. It's like I'm careering down a hill at high speed in a car with no brakes. I must persuade them somehow to allow me something more effective than just talk. I need help urgently.

"Look, if you don't give me something I shall have to self-medicate. I'll have to go to Tesco's and buy myself some tablets. Please help me." I daren't tell them about the bottle in my room.

"Go to the Group, tell them about it."

There's a clear finality about the tone of those words, the repeated message. That is the only thing they're going to suggest. I feel sick with despair. It's utterly hopeless. They don't care about me, they're not going to do anything for me.

Inside me there is a sudden, dramatic change. Well, I'll show them, I seethe inwardly, I'll be all right. I can look after myself. I'll sort this on my own. I don't need their help.

I'm suddenly engulfed by a powerful sensation of certainty that I can deal with this. I already feel stronger knowing that I can make myself feel better, although I'm not yet aware quite how I'm going to do it.

"Fine," I announce in a cold, calm voice that doesn't feel as if it belongs to me. "I'll do what you say. I'm going to Small Group now."

I stand, turn and walk out of the room.

I'm a robot. No emotion. No awareness of my surroundings. I don't have a conscious plan but a strong voice in my head is guiding me. "First go to the water fountain, take some water to your bedroom." I respond obediently.

"Walk up the stairs making sure that you do not attract attention by behaving strangely."

The voice is soothing, comforting, strong…

"Lock your door then open the wardrobe and remove the bottle from its hiding place. Take a handful of the tablets, swallow them with the drink."

This is easy. I feel totally in control now even though my heart is beating too fast because I know I'm doing something that's forbidden. But that makes it exciting too. Gone is the dark emptiness. I feel elated.

"Take some more tablets, don't waste them."

I stare at the blue pills in my hand.

I can't remember how many times I've filled my palm, but there are only four or five left in the bottle.

There's a knock at my door. I jump. The handle moves.

"Polly, why are you in your room? Unlock this door now."

I know if I refuse a member of staff will override the lock.

"Just a minute," I reply quickly.

I down the tablets I'm holding, replace the bottle behind my shoes at the back of the wardrobe.

Opening the door I'm sure that I appear completely normal. One of the nurses is standing there. I recognise her through the mist that is clouding my eyes. I feel sleepy, relaxed. She won't know what's up because I'm not showing any sign of distress. I'll get away with this; she won't know what I've done.

"Have you taken something?" she demands. I don't answer. I find lying difficult.

"What have you taken?"

I remove the brown bottle from its hiding place. She takes it from me.

"Come with me."

"No, I'm going to Group."

I begin the short walk towards the door of the meeting room, which is on the same floor opposite my bedroom.

The nurse has gripped me by the shoulders preventing me from moving.

"You are coming with me. Take care down these stairs." She doesn't let go of my arm.

It seems I don't have a choice. But it doesn't matter. Nothing matters now. I feel warm and fuzzy but I wish these stairs would keep still.

Someone is shouting, "Get an ambulance!"

I'm standing in the entrance supported on either side, I can't resist the blanket of sleepiness covering me, my legs won't support my weight, I'm too heavy, they're giving way…

*

I was on a ventilator for two days, unconscious, unable to breathe for myself. After my discharge from hospital, a week later, I had to deal with the guilt, the shame, the shock…

Apart from my daughter, who spoke willingly about her feelings, the rest of my family made little reference to how my overdose affected them. I am grateful for Rachel's honesty, which is a reflection of the nature of our relationship. It is, undoubtedly, far too painful for the others to vent the anger they must have felt. It wasn't just me that had to deal with the consequences of my massive overdose.

Even now the thought of my close brush with death makes me shudder. If anyone had asked me the day before it happened if I would ever take such a step I would have been horrified at the suggestion. I was sure I had enough insight and awareness not to deal with emotional upheaval in that way.

Now I am constantly on my guard for triggers that could lead to self-destruction. I am more in touch with my feelings. And when I feel in danger I take steps to protect myself like asking Dennis to keep any tablets hidden from me.

Chapter Eleven

Sitting in the psychiatrist's room I'm arguing my case for treatment for my problems, for what has been labelled 'Borderline Personality Disorder' – a term I don't fully understand. Apparently, having a label of some kind makes treatment more likely.

The therapy my psychologist has been requesting for me for the past three years is not locally available, it's only possible on a private basis, which presents an obvious problem. The Health Authority has recently spent thousands of pounds on me for a year's stay in a Therapeutic Community. It was clear to me after a few months that the therapy was not going to work but Marcus urged me to persevere in order to prove my staying power, my ability to stick with it no matter how difficult.

Not surprisingly, the doctor thinks I am unlikely to get funding for further therapy, particularly one that is expensive and privately run. Even my G.P., who has proved so helpful in the past, tells me, "You've been lucky, some people never get any help."

Somehow I have to convince the psychiatrist today to refer me to the panel that decides on how Health Authority money is spent. I have to prove to him that spending a further sum of money on me is likely to be cost-effective. If he isn't convinced he won't even bother to apply.

But the situation doesn't look very hopeful. I come into the category of patients who are ' hard to treat.' And I'm sure he won't have forgotten the incident when I sat in his office refusing to move until he suggested something more effective than yet another prescription for anti-depressants. He has already stated today that he thinks I'm being antagonistic. In my view I am simply repeatedly asking him whether he is going to follow up my psychologist's recommendation that I be referred to the panel. Marcus has written several letters over the years requesting a specific treatment, which he calls Dialectical Behaviour Therapy. A psychologist's opinion does not, however, seem to carry the same weight as a psychiatrist's. Since this doctor is the only person who is in a position to act on my behalf to get it, I feel I need to put some pressure on him. I'm not being offensive, I'm not shouting, I just keep restating my case in the hope that eventually he will acknowledge the urgency.

"What you must understand, Mrs Fielding, is that you are just one among many similar patients waiting for treatment."

I'm sure he's right. But I don't find his statement very helpful. I certainly don't feel he thinks of me as an individual who deserves to be helped. Maybe he hopes I'll just disappear. I feel angry with the system, with him, with the fact that I must fight for myself if I'm to stand any chance of getting the right sort of help. If people like me had a physical disability, one that everyone could see, it might be easier to understand the trauma we endure on a daily basis. Just because our suffering is invisible, does that make us any less entitled to relief from our pain?

I want to run round his room screaming at the top of my voice so that he'll see how outraged, how frustrated I am. But although I feel like it, I'm not a little child and in order to help myself I am going to have to speak in a calm, rational, convincing manner.

After what seems a very long silence I continue, "I need your help, Doctor. I have shown my willingness to keep going in spite of the fact that treatment was not working. I gained insight from it. But it didn't help me to use that insight. I believe that the therapy Marcus is asking for can give me the tools to build the self-esteem and belief in myself that my emotionally and physically abusive upbringing did not give me. And at my age I don't have the luxury of time to wait until this treatment is on offer within County.

"On a conscious level I know I'm an intelligent, creative person with the determination to live a fulfilling, productive life. But subconsciously, the conviction that I am a nobody causes me to be self-destructive. The greater short-term expense of the therapy Marcus suggested would be far outweighed by its long-term benefits and effectiveness for me."

I've tried my best. This feels like an exam I have to pass. I watch the doctor's face closely but there is no discernable expression.

To my utter astonishment he suddenly heaves a long sigh.

"Right, I'll put in an application."

I thank him, walk out of his office relieved that finally something is going to happen. But I can't help thinking about all those of whom I'm simply one, the thousands of others who don't have the resources to fight for themselves, who fall by the wayside, forgotten about by everyone…

*

Recently, my self-destructive thoughts have become constant, compulsive, so difficult not to indulge that I asked the doctor to give me something to help me resist the almost overwhelming temptation to overdose. I have an aversion to taking tablets but I am willing for the present to take the prescribed anti-psychotic mood-altering drugs to keep me on an even keel. I am determined to do whatever it takes to stay alive.

It seems that whenever things are going well I get an enormous impulse to self-sabotage. And lately my life has been good. Dennis and I are going for marriage counselling, we are learning to understand each other's point of view. The children are living busy, positive lives and we have a good relationship with each one of them. And, after months of asking the psychiatrist to get me the treatment I need for my 'Borderline Personality Disorder' I have an appointment in two week's time for an assessment for the new therapy. Marcus continues to support me by talking with me for an hour each week despite the fact that he feels powerless to help me personally on an outpatient basis.

I have an appointment with him today. I begin by telling him about the new tablets. I say I'm having difficulty concentrating.

"That's because they're a chemical cosh," he says. "They dampen down the feelings."

"I hate taking medication. Do you think I should continue with them?"

"They are a better alternative to death."

I begin to cry. " I mustn't give into the temptation to take my life. It would be terrible for the children having to live with the knowledge that their mother committed suicide. I can't, I mustn't do that to them."

He nods.

"Marcus, why has coming to see you never helped me to sort myself out?"

"Because in between our sessions you could never stay focused long enough to do the homework tasks we agreed on."

"Have you heard that I've been turned down by the centre the Health Authority referred me to, the one for self-harmers? I didn't want to go there anyway when I saw the contrast between the magnificent, carefully-tended gardens and the neglected, unwelcoming interior of the building."

"Yes, I know about that. It wouldn't have been the right place for you, but cheaper options for treatment are always the first to be tried. However, rather than talk about that let's concentrate on what's happening now."

"My adoptive mother's voice is always there at the back of my head. Whatever I say to myself that's positive gets thrown out because at the core of my being I don't believe it."

"In my view your adoptive mother manipulated

you to get rid of her own negative feelings. She was one of those people who are somehow able to make another person feel as bad as themselves. She built you up by getting you to tell her the good things you'd done, like getting excellent grades in your schoolwork, so that she could dismiss them, and make you feel bad. The worst feeling she instilled in you was shame. Research has shown that once a child has been made to feel shame, the rest is easy. Your mother then had you right where she wanted and could play about with your feelings."

"But why me, why not Rita or Teresa?"

"Well, Rita was her own daughter so that might have been more difficult and perhaps Teresa put up some resistance. Anyway, by the time Teresa came along she already had you thoroughly trained to respond to her in the way she wanted."

"Perhaps she wasn't aware of what she was doing." I'm past taking responsibility for her actions but I want to find some excuse for what she did.

"She was compulsively driven but at some level she knew exactly what was she was up to. She couldn't fail to see the disappointment in your eyes, she heard the distress in your voice and noticed the tears rolling down your face."

I can't believe what he's telling me.. Much as I respect Marcus, he must be wrong. He didn't know my Mummy, she couldn't have deliberately, knowingly inflicted such unbearable pain on me. I decide to change the subject.

"What about Daddy?"

"He didn't protect you. And perhaps the thrashings were his way of venting his feelings about his marriage."

"But that's cruel! How could anyone do that to a child?"

Marcus looks at me; shrugs his shoulders. Obviously he can't understand it either.

He leans towards me, an earnest expression on his face.

"Your mother may have dismissed your efforts. But there is something I have to tell you which you may choose to discount. In my experience it is extremely rare for someone who's been abused to do what you have done with your children. Despite your background you have recognised and acknowledged their achievements and valued them for themselves. That doesn't happen very often. Usually the abusive cycle continues. You have managed to break it."

I think about the beautiful, positive individuals he's referring to. I'd like to think he's right.

After a pause I continue, "What about Dialectical Behaviour Therapy? What does it involve?"

"It's residential and it's training to cope with difficult emotions and social interaction whilst giving ongoing support to practice the methods they teach. You already have a great deal of insight into your problems but it's wasted unless you learn how to make use of it. However, the good news is that funding has been approved."

I feel a momentary sense of relief before the familiar panic begins. "What if they don't accept me? What if they turn me away?"

"You want certainty and I can't give you that. I've presented a very strong case and all I can suggest is that you show them yourself; you don't need to lose control but don't hide your feelings. Be emotionally present like you are today."

With that parting advice the session is over.

I walk out of Marcus's room with a more positive outlook. I've got a warm glow inside from his praise. And every step from now is on the road to recovery. I know I am going to have to work hard, that progress is up to me. The next therapy is going to help because this time I shall be taking responsibility for the process rather than allowing it to be done to me. Even if there are setbacks on the way I am determined reach my goals of emotional well-being and a life worth living.

And Finally…

Inevitably, an abusive childhood has an enormous, enduring impact. And its effects depend on personality. Some people are able to rise above what has happened to them. They learn to value themselves and lead productive, highly successful lives. Others may react by turning to drugs, alcohol, crime…

Inability to deal with the past may result in eating disorders, depression, phobias, obsessions…

And there are those who appear confident, coping and high achievers whilst inwardly struggling daily with their demons. Like them, for many years I remained firmly stuck in my past. Only recently did I reach the point where I was truly ready to discard the familiarity of my inward negative state, despite the frightening uncertainty of change.

Just as someone will only give up smoking when they take a conscious decision to do it, so resolving emotional problems first requires self-awareness, then a firm decision to make the necessary changes, however painful.

Accepting that the past cannot be changed is crucial to recovery. We can do nothing to alter what has happened to us but we can take control of the present and influence the future. It is essential to let the past go and move on, making sure that we get the best possible help to do so.

Working as a teacher and having my own children helped soothe my pain. Helping to build the self-esteem of children, watching them thrive as I praised their efforts, seeing them emerge as beautiful people in their own right because I loved them for who they were, gave me something I was denied.

Getting absorbed in an activity can be an extremely helpful respite from seemingly unsolvable problems. I have spent many hours immersed in writing, producing pastel pictures, giving massages, playing the piano... Some of the greatest music, art and literary works have been the products of disturbed minds!

Others may choose to take up a hobby like gardening, going to the gym, photography, chess, jigsaw puzzles...

But ultimately, there is no one solution. Everyone must find a route that is right for them.

Some readers of this book will have been able to identify with, and hopefully express, many of the emotions I felt compelled to put onto paper. I hope this has given them the knowledge that they are not alone.

There is a pressing need for greater input of resources to our mental health system. Medication and locked doors are not enough.

CPSIA information can be obtained at www.ICGtesting.com
Printed in the USA
LVOW12s2101050514

384498LV00033B/1395/P